FOURTH
EDITION

Legal, Ethical, and Practical Aspects of
PATIENT CARE DOCUMENTATION

A Guide for Rehabilitation Professionals

RONALD W. SCOTT, PT, JD, EDD, LLM, MSBA

Attorney-Mediator and Clinical Consultant
Cibolo, Texas

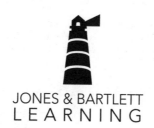

JONES & BARTLETT
LEARNING

World Headquarters
Jones & Bartlett Learning
5 Wall Street
Burlington, MA 01803
978-443-5000
info@jblearning.com
www.jblearning.com

Jones & Bartlett Learning books and products are available through most bookstores and online booksellers. To contact Jones & Bartlett Learning directly, call 800-832-0034, fax 978-443-8000, or visit our website, www.jblearning.com.

Substantial discounts on bulk quantities of Jones & Bartlett Learning publications are available to corporations, professional associations, and other qualified organizations. For details and specific discount information, contact the special sales department at Jones & Bartlett Learning via the above contact information or send an email to specialsales@jblearning.com.

Production Credits
Publisher: David D. Cella
Acquisitions Editor: Katey Birtcher
Managing Editor: Maro Gartside
Editorial Assistant: Teresa Reilly, Kayla Dos Santos
Senior Production Editor: Renée Sekerak
Production Assistant: Sean Coombs
Marketing Manager: Grace Richards
Manufacturing and Inventory Control Supervisor: Amy Bacus
Composition: Laserwords Private Limited, Chennai, India
Cover Design: Scott Moden
Cover Images: A doctor and a nurse using laptops © John Wollwerth/ShutterStock, Inc.; Woman strapping leg © AbleStock; A physical therapist holds a model of the bones of the hand while speaking to a patient © Photodisc; Man using hand grip © AbleStock
Printing and Binding: Edwards Brothers Malloy
Cover Printing: Edwards Brothers Malloy

Library of Congress Cataloging-in-Publication Data
Scott, Ronald W.
  Legal, ethical, and practical aspects of patient care documentation : a guide for rehabilitation professionals / Ron Scott. — 4th ed.
    p. ; cm.
  Rev. ed. of: Legal aspects of documenting patient care for rehabilitation professionals / Ronald W. Scott. 3rd ed. c2006.
  Includes bibliographical references and index.
  ISBN 978-0-7637-9910-6 (pbk.)
  1. Medical records—Law and legislation—United States. 2. Medical care—Law and legislation—United States. 3. Medical records—Management. I. Scott, Ronald W. Legal aspects of documenting patient care for rehabilitation professionals. II. Title.
  [DNLM: 1. Forms and Records Control—legislation & jurisprudence—United States. 2. Forms and Records Control—methods—United States. 3. Medical Records—legislation & jurisprudence—United States. 4. Quality Assurance, Health Care—legislation & jurisprudence—United States. 5. Rehabilitation—organization & administration—United States. W 32.5 AA1]
  KF3827.R4S385 2013
  344.7304′1—dc23
                                                                        2011031272

6048
Printed in the United States of America
17 16 15 14 13   10 9 8 7 6 5 4 3 2

I dedicate this book with love and gratitude to my wife of 38+ years, Pepi Barba Scott, without whose love and support my many life projects would not have come to fruition. I also dedicate this work to my three darling grandchildren —Isabel, Jonas, and Marlee. Abuela and abuelo love you!

Contents

Preface

The healthcare delivery system is increasingly complex. As care delivery and patient care documentation become more streamlined with improved technology, healthcare providers and organizations must strive to maintain an empathetic human face on the services we provide, because patients come to us vulnerable, frightened about their conditions, and trusting in us as their fiduciaries.

Patient care documentation epitomizes the best in clinical healthcare delivery by placing our work product directly and prominently in the public eye. The "stories" that unravel from patient care documentation—whether in paper or electronic format—are the narratives of how millions of lives are heroically saved or made better every year through our efforts.

With great power comes great responsibility. Healthcare professionals hold the very lives of their patients in their hands every day, and because of that level of power and responsibility, are held to the highest ethical and legal standards of any professionals on Earth. There is perhaps no nobler calling than to dedicate oneself to the optimization of patients' health and well-being, and, indirectly, that of their families and significant others and society-at-large.

This book is written with the intention of providing a roadmap to health professionals and students about the panoply of issues surrounding patient care documentation. From practical to ethical to legal intricacies of documenting what we do for patients, I hope to provide basic guidance—in nonlegalese terms—about how to meet your documentation-related duties to patients and also to yourselves, in order to minimize healthcare malpractice liability exposure.

This book contains six chapters. Chapter 1, *Patient Care Documentation Within the Legal Environment*, presents an overview of the law of healthcare malpractice and its relationship to patient care documentation and other forms of health professional communication. Chapter 2, *Clinical Patient Care Documentation Methods and Management*, overviews the nature, contents, formats, and processes of healthcare clinical patient care documentation. Chapter 2 includes 25 documentation problems, errors, and suggestions. Chapter 3, *The Patient Care Record in Legal Proceedings*, focuses on the patient care record as a business and legal document, and examines its uses in administrative and legal proceedings. Chapter 4, *Patient Care Record Informed Consent Documentation Issues*, examines the concept of patient informed consent, as it relates to healthcare examination, intervention, an documentation. Chapter 5, *Patient Care Documentation and Clinical Quality-Risk Management Programs and Initiatives*, examines the processes of patient care-related quality and liability risk management. Chapter 6, *Current Issues in Patient Care Documentation*, presents a summary of selected important patient care documentation issues that providers encounter in everyday clinical practice.

Each chapter contains cases, exercises, and a Focus on Ethics vignette for review. Each chapter also ends with a references and readings list for further study.

I hope that the information presented in this book helps you to better serve patients under your care, and to have greater peace of mind while doing so. Best wishes for continued practice success!

Ron Scott, JD, EdD, PT

Acknowledgments

I wish to acknowledge all of the dedicated healthcare clinical and support professionals who work tirelessly and selflessly to better the lives and well-being of patients under our care. Thanks, too, to the editorial staff at Jones & Bartlett Learning for their diligent support and patience in helping me to bring this book to fruition.

About the Author

Ron Scott began his career as a healthcare professional in 1969 and has been an attorney since 1983. While working as a university professor from 1985 to the present, by 1990 his expertise expanded into writing, editing, mediating interpersonal disputes, and being a writers' coach.

After a tour of duty during the Vietnam War as a Navy hospital corpsman and operating room technician, Ron attended the University of Pittsburgh's Physical Therapy Program, and graduated a McMillan Scholar and Jessie Wright awardee. He went on to earn six other academic degrees, including his MA in Spanish (Millersville University), MSPT (Samuel Merritt College), MSBA (Boston University), JD (University of San Diego), EdD (University of Texas, Austin), and LLM (Judge Advocate General's School).

Ron was a civilian and Army physical therapist and clinical manager for a decade. For six years, he was an Army JAG Corp attorney specializing in criminal prosecution and defense, and healthcare malpractice claims settlement.

After completing his military career as a Major in the Army Medical Specialist Corps, Ron became an associate professor and interim chair in physical therapy at the University of Texas Health Science Center, San Antonio, where he now teaches Electrophysical Agents, Ethics, Management, and Medical Spanish. He is also currently a faculty member in six other programs: Husson University (physical therapy), Rocky Mountain University of Health Sciences (nursing, physical and occupational therapy, and allied health), the University of Indianapolis (occupational and physical therapy), the University of Montana and University of South Florida (transitional doctor of physical therapy), and Webster University (graduate business programs).

Ron also currently works as an attorney-mediator, specializing in employment, family, and health law. This is his 13th book.

Reviewers

Karen Coupe, PT, DPT, MSEd
Faculty
Physical Therapy Assistant Program
Keiser University
Ft. Lauderdale, FL

Les R. Schmeltz, AuD
Assistant Professor
Audiology
A.T. Still University
Mesa, AZ

Barbara Banning, MEd, OTR/L
Program Director
Occupational Therapy Assistant Program
Augusta Technical College
Augusta, GA

Lora L. Davis, PT, DPT
Physical Therapy
A.T. Still University
Mesa, AZ

CHAPTER 1

Patient Care Documentation Within the Legal Environment

This introductory chapter presents an overview of the law of health-care malpractice and its relationship to patient care documentation and other forms of professional communication, focusing on the following concepts: the legal bases for imposing healthcare malpractice liability on healthcare providers and organizations, professional negligence and the legal standard of care, depositions, expert witness testimony, patient abandonment, and judicial and legislative tort reform initiatives designed to dampen the incidence of healthcare malpractice claims and lawsuits. This chapter—like the remaining chapters—includes case examples and one or more Focus on Ethics vignettes. The material in this and in succeeding chapters explains in straightforward language how to minimize liability exposure through effective patient care documentation.

THE HEALTHCARE MALPRACTICE CRISIS

In the last four decades, the United States (expanding more recently to other nations) has experienced what has been labeled a healthcare "malpractice crisis," characterized by a public perception of increasing numbers of legal actions and larger civil malpractice verdicts in favor of patient-plaintiffs and against defendant-healthcare providers and organizations. This phenomenon has affected the practice not only of medicine, but of every primary healthcare discipline that provides direct patient care services, including: advanced clinical nurse practitioners and nurse anesthetists, physical and occupational therapists, physician assistants, and other primary healthcare professionals.

Primary healthcare providers face a high degree of malpractice exposure, not only because they treat patients when they are most vulnerable and at risk—sick or injured and often in pain—but also because of many other factors. External factors that increase providers' malpractice exposure include a greater sense of consumerism among the patient population, intensified federal and state regulation of healthcare delivery, and a metamorphosis in the healthcare milieu away from informal, time-intensive, personalized care in favor of increasingly competitive, rapid, "business-like" delivery of healthcare services to patients.

Some primary healthcare disciplines, including, for example, physical therapy, have undergone substantive internal professional changes that may increase their members' healthcare malpractice liability risk exposure. Some internal factors that may create greater legal risks for providers within these disciplines specifically include: expanding scope and breadth of professional practice; the increasing importance, utilization, and highly visible presence of these professions within the healthcare delivery system; the trends toward direct-access practice or practice without physician referral in more and more jurisdictions; clinical specialty certification; and the publication of practice guidelines, such as *The Guide to Physical Therapist Practice*. Note that few, if any, other healthcare disciplines have created similar comprehensive practice guides because of justifiable fear, despite any disclaimers to the contrary, that patient-plaintiff attorneys will attempt to use, and courts will allow their use, in healthcare malpractice proceedings to help fact-finders (juries and judges) understand the complex legal standard of care.

Obviously, not all healthcare malpractice claims and legal actions are frivolous. There are a substantial number of medical mistakes annually that result in serious bodily injury to, or the death of, patients. The Institute of Medicine (IOM), a Washington, D.C.-based nongovernmental organization focused on health, reported in 1999 that approximately 100,000 such medical mistakes adversely affect hospitalized patients per year. In 2004, HealthGrades, a Colorado-based private entity that assesses and publicly reports on the quality of healthcare delivery provided by hospitals, long-term care facilities, and physicians, doubled the Institute's previous estimate of annual inpatient medical mistakes to approximately 200,000. The 2005 Harvard Leape study reiterated the findings of the IOM when it concluded that there are approximately 100,000 annual inpatient deaths in the United States from preventable medical mistakes. A 2006 IOM report concluded that medication errors account for most of the 1.5 million patient injuries per year attributable to medical mistakes. Although not all medical mistakes constitute healthcare malpractice—some, for instance, may be attributable to non-negligent provider errors in clinical judgment or the patients' own contributory negligence—many do.

Healthcare malpractice plaintiffs do not prevail in their legal cases as often as they lose. On average, patient-plaintiffs prevail in their lawsuits against healthcare providers less than half of the time. A 2001 study conducted by the United States Department of Justice found that in the 75 largest counties in the United States, patient-plaintiffs won healthcare malpractice cases only 27 percent of the time. By 2005, there were only 14,033 healthcare malpractice case payments from settlements or court judgments nationwide, down 15.4 percent from 16,588 in 2001, according to Public Citizen's Congress Watch. The median jury verdict in medical malpractice cases in 2009 was $1,018.86, according to Jury Verdict Research.

Healthcare professionals and clinical managers can do many things in practice to minimize the incidence of claims of healthcare malpractice and malpractice lawsuits. Of paramount importance is excellence in communications between healthcare providers and patients and among healthcare providers who treat patients. In communicating with patients, providers must remember to explain in simple layperson's terms what they are doing during clinical examinations. Providers must similarly explain examination and diagnostic test results to patients (or surrogate decision-makers) in simple layperson's language. Patients not only want information about their health status and care but are entitled to it as a universal ethical and legal principle and fundamental human right. Under the mixed ethical-legal concept of informed consent, healthcare providers must convey to patients sufficient information about their health status to allow patients to make informed choices about whether to accept or decline recommended interventions. (Keep in mind that *all* proposed therapeutic interventions are recommended, not directed.) Effective clinical documentation of primary provider–patient communication processes, especially concerning informed disclosure and consent, is crucial to managing malpractice risk exposure.

In addition to effective communication with patients, healthcare providers must also communicate effectively and systematically with other healthcare professionals who are either concurrently treating a given patient or who will treat that patient in the future. The principal means of communicating information among healthcare providers is through patient care documentation. Accurate, timely, thorough, and concise documentation can be the deciding factor for whether a patient lives or dies. Effective documentation also has "professional" life-and-death consequences for healthcare providers charged with malpractice. In a malpractice trial, tried perhaps many years after care was rendered, what is written in the treatment record may constitute the only objective evidence of whether care given to a patient-plaintiff by a malpractice health professional-defendant met or breached minimally acceptable practice standards. While a defense attorney at trial may be able to dispel the inference that if something "wasn't documented, it wasn't done," proof by legal standards that care *was* rendered to a patient, and rendered appropriately and within the legal standard of care, is most easily facilitated through accurate, timely, thorough, and concise patient care documentation by responsible primary healthcare professionals.

Lopopolo reported that effective communication is the most important LAMP (leadership, administration, management, and professionalism) skill that a primary healthcare professional requires in order to be successful in clinical practice. In its 2006 physical therapy malpractice claims study, CNA reported that the failure to timely communicate vital patient information to other primary healthcare providers having a need to know is the most severe (costly) type of physical therapist malpractice claim it processes. CNA reported that the average indemnity (payout) for failure-to-communicate physical therapist malpractice claims was $277,425.

Consider the following hypothetical case example: A is a supervisory physical therapist; B is A's physical therapist assistant, working with patient C, who is postoperative day 6, right knee arthroscopy. C has made little progress in achieving full functional active range of motion of the right knee. In fact, C's active range of motion decreased from 25/75 on day 3 post-op to 27/70 on day 6. A directs B to write an urgent progress note, apprizing D, C's orthopedic surgeon on this fact and seeking guidance on how best to proceed. By the end of the Friday work day (when progress notes are written), B forgets to write the progress note on C. By Monday, C's right knee active range of motion has further decreased to 40/60, totally impeding C's gait and necessitating a costly manipulation under anesthesia the same afternoon.

In a malpractice claim for professional negligence, who is liable to C, and why? What documentation strategy would have prevented this adverse event?

A and B are both liable to C for professional negligence, or substandard care delivery. As licensed health professionals, A and B have fiduciary and legal duties to act reasonably and in C's best health interests, which both failed to do. A is legally vicariously (indirectly) responsible as a supervisor for B's patient care documentation.

The optimal approach to meet legal and fiduciary duties in this case would have been for B to write the urgent progress note immediately (assuming that B is privileged under state law and facility policy to do so), and have it checked and countersigned by A. A then should have immediately followed up the urgent notation with a phone call or instant text message to communicate directly with surgeon D.

Besides effective communication and documentation, other strategies can be used to help lessen the risk of malpractice actions. These include simple things such as treating patients with empathy and compassion; practicing only within one's personal scope of clinical competence and within the legal parameters of one's professional state practice act; consulting with other healthcare providers whenever necessary; and establishing within healthcare facilities effective, proactive quality and liability risk management programs to monitor and evaluate patient care activities, including establishing appropriate patient care documentation standards, and to minimize malpractice risk exposure.

Reflective of the expanding domain of primary healthcare practice, legal issues concerning physical therapy and other nonphysician healthcare specialties have received greater attention by legal and healthcare authors in the recent past. Along with private education entities, professional associations, including, among others, the American Health Lawyers Association, the American Medical Association, the American Nurses Association, the American Occupational Therapy Association, and the American Physical Therapy Association, are sponsoring more professional seminars on selected legal topics such as liability risk management, expert testimony, the legal standard of care, and HIPAA compliance, among other relevant topics.

Focus on Ethics

A is an orthopedic surgeon who has just completed right knee arthroscopic surgery on patient B. It is a Friday afternoon, past the end of the normal workday, and A does not write a postoperative therapy order or orally communicate with physical therapy about the need to commence intervention for patient B on Saturday morning. As a result, B's care is unnecessarily delayed until Monday late morning. Which of the four biomedical ethical principles (beneficence [acting in patients' best interests], nonmaleficence [do no malicious intentional harm], respect for patient autonomy [self-determination], or justice) was violated by one or more health professionals in this vignette? What systematic processes might prevent such errors in the future?

(See Suggested Answer Framework in Appendix D.)

MALPRACTICE DEFINED

Legal writers and scholars have used two approaches to defining healthcare malpractice. Under the traditional approach, the definition of healthcare malpractice includes only conduct that constitutes professional negligence: the overwhelming basis for imposition of malpractice liability. Under a broader approach, however, every potential legal basis for imposition of healthcare malpractice liability, including professional negligence, breach of a therapeutic contractual promise made by a provider to a patient, patient or client injury from dangerously defective care-related equipment or other products (strict product liability), strict (absolute, nonfault-based) liability for abnormally dangerous care-related activities, and patient or client injury that results from intentional provider misconduct in the course of patient care, may be included in the definition. Defective or incomplete patient care documentation may constitute either professional negligence or intentional misconduct, depending on the circumstances surrounding the case.

Most of the earlier referenced bases of malpractice liability—negligence, intentional conduct, and product and strict liability—are classified as *torts* (French for "wrongs"), a class of legal actions that encompasses most personal injuries except those caused by breach of contract. Torts are classified as *private actions* because they involve injuries personal to private parties, in contrast to *crimes*, which are public actions, or wrongs against society as a whole.

Two Formulations for the Definition of "Healthcare Malpractice"

Traditional narrow definition: Professional (care-related) negligence only

Broad definition (trend): Any potential legal basis for imposition of liability, including:

- Professional negligence
- Breach of a patient–professional contractual promise
- Liability for defective care-related equipment or products that injure patients or clients
- Strict liability (absolute liability without regard for fault) for abnormally dangerous care-related professional activities
- Intentional care-related provider misconduct

The broad definition of healthcare malpractice is superior to the traditional definition in several respects. From a risk-management perspective, its inclusiveness helps to focus the attention of healthcare system and organizational managers, educators, and clinicians on more parameters than just professional negligence. Also, it serves to make everyone in the healthcare system aware of the fact that the legal system exists to protect the most widely variegated range of rights of patients and clients.

Professional negligence, breach of contract, and intentional misconduct are all fault-based bases for liability. That is, each requires a finding of some degree of culpability on the part of the defendant-healthcare provider for the plaintiff to prevail. On the other hand, product liability and strict liability for abnormally dangerous activities are non-fault-based, meaning that no culpability need be established for a finding of liability against a defendant. For these last two bases of liability, like vicarious (indirect) liability discussed later in the chapter, a judge or jury awards a verdict against a defendant as a matter of social policy. The operative question in such cases often is, "Between two innocent parties, who best can bear the burden of financial responsibility?"

PROFESSIONAL NEGLIGENCE

Professional negligence by healthcare providers involves delivery of patient care that falls below the standards expected of ordinary reasonable practitioners of the same profession acting under the same or similar circumstances. By definition, professional negligence involves care that falls below the minimal acceptable standards for practice, or substandard care. To be professionally negligent means that the provider did or failed to do something in the course of patient history-taking, examination, evaluation, intervention, referral, or follow-up that other, similarly situated healthcare professionals would not accept as constituting minimally acceptable care. Put still another way, professional negligence is legally actionable carelessness. Negligent substandard patient care documentation by a provider, when it causes patient injury, constitutes legally actionable professional negligence-based healthcare malpractice.

Whether care is negligent is usually determined at trial by expert testimony by one or more professional peers. To qualify as an expert, such a witness must be familiar with the following: (1) the care-related process or procedure at issue in the case, and (2) the standard of care for the defendant-healthcare provider's discipline in the relevant geographical frame of reference at the time that care and alleged patient injury took place.

Qualifications of an Expert Witness Testifying on the Legal Standard of Care

In-depth knowledge of the following:

- The healthcare examination, evaluative, or intervention-related issue in the case
- The applicable standard of care at the time that care was rendered

A patient suing a healthcare professional for malpractice must prove the following four elements at trial: (1) The healthcare provider owed the patient a professional duty of care; (2) The provider violated or breached the duty owed; (3) The violation of the standard of care caused physical and/or mental injury to the patient; (4) As a result, the patient is entitled to money "damages" to make the patient as whole again as possible.

The standard (or burden) of proof for proving each of these required elements in civil malpractice trials is "preponderance of the evidence," which equates to "more likely than not" that the trier of fact (jury, or judge acting as fact-finder when there is no jury in the case) believes that the patient-plaintiff's evidence presented at trial is more credible than that of the health professional-defendant.

The Four Requisite Elements of Proof for a Patient-Plaintiff in a Healthcare Malpractice Trial

1. The provider owed the patient a special duty of care.

2. The provider violated the special duty owed.

3. As a result, the patient was injured.

4. The patient is entitled to legally recognized money damages.

ORDINARY NEGLIGENCE VERSUS PROFESSIONAL NEGLIGENCE

Many clinical situations involving patient injury do not involve professional negligence, but only ordinary or general negligence. Ordinary negligence, even when it occurs in the healthcare clinical setting, does not constitute healthcare malpractice.

A common form of ordinary or general negligence involves what is termed *premises liability*. From falling on a slippery floor surface to being run into by a wheelchair or stretcher to being struck by an ambulance while walking in front of a hospital, ordinary premises negligence involves the kinds of injury-causing events that can occur in any physical setting—from a retail store to a college or university to a public street or sidewalk. Ordinary negligence, then, is not healthcare malpractice, as it is not directly care-related. For that reason, with ordinary negligence, an injured patient usually need not introduce expert testimony to attempt to show a breach of the professional standard of care, because everyday situations such as slips and falls are within the common knowledge of lay jurors, who thus do not need experts to explain the mechanism of injury to them.

THE PROFESSIONAL STANDARD OF CARE

When cases do involve allegations of professional negligence, the plaintiff must usually establish the applicable standard of care and its breach by the defendant-healthcare provider. There are three different formulations of the standard of care in effect in various jurisdictions in the United States. Under the traditional view, healthcare professionals are compared with reasonably competent peers practicing only in the exact same community. This standard originally was applied to prevent prejudicing rural healthcare providers who lacked comparable access to the modern technology and resources available to urban-based colleagues. Modernly, this standard is no longer applicable.

The current majority rule is to compare a defendant-healthcare professional with reasonably competent peers practicing in either the same or similar communities. In one reported physical therapy malpractice case, *Novey v. Kishawakee Community Health Services*, the court ruled that an occupational therapist lacked legal competence to testify about whether a physical therapist met or breached the standard of care, because occupational therapy and physical therapy are different "schools of medicine." This case's legal holding potentially has broad implications for healthcare professionals attempting to testify for or against healthcare professional-litigants of different disciplines on the litigant-professional's legal standard of care. (The extent of influence of the *Novey* decision on future cases depends on whether state or federal judges in cases outside of the state choose to adopt the decision as precedent. State court judges hearing cases outside the state in which a case is heard are not bound by law to follow the decision reached.)

The trend regarding the standard of care is to apply a statewide or nationwide standard to all health professionals of a given discipline and compare a defendant charged with healthcare malpractice with reasonably competent peers acting under the same or similar circumstances, without regard to geographical limitations. Courts (by case law) and legislatures (by statute) are imposing this standard more and more, because of standardization of education and training and because of advances in communications technology that remove earlier disadvantages of rural or isolated practitioners. The standard of care for board-certified clinical specialists is also a uniform national standard of care.

Three Formulations for the Legal Standard of Care for Healthcare Professionals

The three formulations for the legal standard of healthcare clinical practice all compare the defendant in a healthcare malpractice case with reasonably competent peers and ask whether such a peer would or could reasonably have acted like the defendant under the same or similar circumstances as existed in a pending lawsuit. The three formulations differ only in their geographical frame of reference.

1. *Traditional rule:* Compare defendant with peers in the exact same community.

2. *Modern majority rule:* Compare defendant with peers in the same community or in similar communities, statewide, or nationwide.

3. *Trend:* Compare defendant with any or all peers, statewide or nationwide, acting under the same or similar circumstances.

RES IPSA LOQUITUR: INFERENCES AND PRESUMPTIONS OF HEALTH PROFESSIONAL NEGLIGENCE

Occasionally, a healthcare malpractice plaintiff will be unable, for reasons beyond the plaintiff's control, to prove that care-related injuries were caused by a breach of the duty of professional care by the defendant. For example, a comatose patient who is injured during surgery cannot testify about the cause of the injuries. Under such circumstances, courts may permit negligence to be inferred, or require it to be presumed by a jury, against a healthcare professional-defendant, under a legal principle called *res ipsa loquitur* (Latin for "the thing [i.e., the patient's injury] speaks for itself").

If negligence is merely inferable, a jury is free to infer negligence against the defendant or not, at its will. If, however, negligence must be legally presumed, then the burden shifts to the defendant to produce sufficient evidence to rebut the presumption of negligence in order to avoid the imposition of liability. For example, assume hypothetically that a comatose patient sustained a broken femur during or about the time that a defendant-registered nurse administered passive range of motion. If, under *res ipsa loquitur*, negligence is to be inferred, the jury deciding the case is free to disregard the inference, irrespective of whether the nurse's attorney puts forward evidence in an attempt to rebut or counter the inference of negligence. If, however, negligence is ordered by the judge to be presumed, a formal legal burden shifts from the plaintiff to the nurse's counsel to introduce sufficient evidence to rebut the presumption of negligence. Such evidence might consist of testimony of a radiologist who read the patient's radiographs while the patient was an inpatient (called a fact, or percipient, witness) that the patient suffered from severe osteoporosis, which might have caused the femoral fracture.

For the doctrine of *res ipsa loquitur* to apply and relieve the plaintiff of carrying the sole legal burden of production of evidence in a case, three factors must be present. First, the plaintiff's injuries must be the type that normally do not happen absent negligence (carelessness) on somebody's part. Second, the defendant-healthcare provider must have exercised exclusive control over the instrumentality that caused the plaintiff's injuries. Finally, the plaintiff must not have been contributorily negligent in causing the injury in issue.

One reported physical therapy malpractice case, *Greater Southeast Community Hospital Foundation v. Walker*, concerned a patient burned by a moist heat pack. In that case, the trial court allowed an inference of negligence under *res ipsa loquitur*. On appeal, the court reversed (disallowed) the verdict at the trial level in favor of the patient, because testimony at trial had raised a question as to whether the patient had manipulated the moist heat pack during treatment. With such a question unresolved, it was ruled that it was improper to invoke *res ipsa loquitur*, because the moist heat pack might not have been under the therapist's exclusive control, but also under the patient's control, and the patient might have been contributorily negligent for having manipulated the moist heat pack.

Res Ipsa Loquitur: When Negligence Is Inferred or Presumed Without Proof by the Patient

1. The patient's injury was the kind that normally does not occur absent negligence.

2. The defendant-healthcare provider exercised exclusive control over the medication, modality, or treatment that caused injury to the patient.

3. The patient did not contribute in any way to causing his or her own injury.

DEFENSES TO HEALTHCARE MALPRACTICE ACTIONS

Two important defenses available to defendant-healthcare professionals, among many others, are the statute of limitations and comparative fault. The former is a procedural defense (also known as a legal *technicality*), and the latter is a substantive defense.

Statutes of Limitations

Statutes of limitations are legislatively enacted laws in effect in every state that limit the time period within which a private plaintiff in a civil case, or a prosecutor in a criminal case, may commence a lawsuit. There are often special rules applicable to healthcare malpractice, which vary from state to state. Generally, though, the "time clock" begins to run against a patient when the patient discovers or reasonably should have discovered that he or she was injured and knows the source (but not necessarily the cause) of the injury. The running of statutes of limitations may be interrupted or *tolled* by such factors as continuous treatment by a defendant-provider, infancy (where the patient has not reached the age of majority), or mental incapacitation of a plaintiff. Many states, however, as part of recent tort reform, have followed the more absolute federal standard, which sets a firm two-year statute of limitations from the date of injury for initiating malpractice legal actions, irrespective of any factors or excuses.

One reported physical therapy case, *Myer v. Woodall*, concerned different statutes of limitations in effect in the state of the lawsuit for professional and ordinary negligence. What resulted was the patient, who was allegedly injured while being transported to physical therapy, was held to have the right to sue the aide who transported the patient to physical therapy but not the physical therapist or the hospital, because the professional statute of limitations had expired. The phenomenon of shortened statutes of limitations for healthcare malpractice actions, like statutes of repose, is a result of tort reform legislation designed to curb the number of healthcare malpractice legal actions.

Comparative Fault

Another major defense in healthcare malpractice legal actions is comparative fault. Comparative fault involves consideration by a judge or jury, not just of a healthcare professional-defendant's conduct, but also that of the patient-plaintiff. Under comparative fault principles, a defendant's liability may be reduced, or eliminated altogether, if the plaintiff violated the expected standard of reasonable care for his or her own safety. There are two formulations for assessing a plaintiffs fault. In contributory negligence jurisdictions, a plaintiff 's case is dismissed and the plaintiff has no legal remedy if he or she was in any way contributorily negligent in causing his or her injuries—even one percent or less at fault. Because this "all-or-nothing" rule is so harsh, it has been subject to many exceptions, such as who had the "last clear chance" to prevent patient-plaintiff injury. It is not currently the law in the overwhelming majority of states.

Most states use comparative negligence as their rule when assessing a plaintiff 's conduct. In most states using comparative negligence, a plaintiff may still prevail in a legal case if he or she was either (depending on the jurisdiction) less than 50 percent at fault or 50 percent or less at fault. A few comparative negligence states allow a plaintiff to recover irrespective of degree of fault. This concept is called *pure* comparative negligence. In a pure comparative negligence state, a patient who was 90 percent at fault for his or her own injuries and who sustained $2 million in damages might still recover $200,000 (10 percent of $2 million).

VICARIOUS LIABILITY

Vicarious liability addresses (in addition to partnership liability) circumstances under which an employer, such as a healthcare organization or system, bears indirect legal and financial responsibility for the conduct of a person, such as an employee. The concept of vicarious liability dates back to medieval times and, in legal circles, is often referred to by its Latin name, *respondeat superior* ("let the master answer").

Employer Vicarious Liability

The basic rule of vicarious liability is that an employer is indirectly liable for the job-related conduct of an employee when the wrongdoer (*tortfeasor*) is acting within the scope of his or her employment at the time the negligence occurred. Therefore, when a hospital-based primary healthcare provider is alleged to have committed professional negligence or care-related intentional misconduct (such as sexual battery) while treating a patient, the hospital employing the provider may be required to pay a money judgment if the provider's negligence or intentional misconduct is proven in court.

An employer's indirect responsibility for an employee's negligence does not excuse the individual provider who actually committed the negligence from financial responsibility. The tortfeasor is always personally responsible for the consequences of his or her own conduct. The concept of vicarious liability, however, gives the tort victim another party (usually with more available assets) to make a claim against or to sue. When an employer is required to pay a settlement or judgment for the negligence of an employee, the employer then has the legal right to seek indemnification from the employee for this monetary outlay.

Is it fair to impose liability on an employer who is innocent of any wrongdoing? In balancing the considerations between an innocent patient-victim and an equally innocent employer, the legal system weighs in favor of the patient. There are several good reasons for this. First, it is the employer, not the patient, who is best equipped to control the quality of care rendered by its healthcare providers. Second, the employer earns revenue from the official activities of its employees and contractors and should, therefore, bear responsibility for the activities that generate such revenue. Third, the employer is better able to bear the risk of financial loss—through economic loss allocation (e.g., purchasing liability insurance and establishing prices for health professional services) as part of the cost of doing business.

An employer may be held vicariously liable for wrongdoing by others who are not employees. In the relatively few cases addressing the issue, courts also have imposed vicarious liability on hospitals for the negligence of volunteers, equating unpaid volunteers with employees. For this reason, hospitals and clinics using the services of volunteers should carry liability insurance for volunteers' activities and include them in orientation to relevant policies and procedures, including workplace safety measures.

Partnership Vicarious Liability

Another area of vicarious liability involves general partnerships, wherein each partner is considered to be the legal agent of the other partner. Absent an unambiguous express agreement to the contrary, each partner normally is vicariously liable or indirectly financially responsible for the other partners' negligent acts or omissions committed within the scope of activities of the partnership.

Exceptions to Vicarious Liability

Intentional Misconduct

There are several important exceptions to vicarious liability. Although an employer may be liable for employees' negligence, the employer may not be legally responsible for unforeseeable intentional misconduct committed by its employees. An example of such unforeseeable intentional misconduct in the healthcare setting might include the commission of sexual battery on a patient by an emergency room security guard or by another patient. (Such conclusions about vicarious liability are acutely case-specific and involve considerations of whether the employer undertook all available reasonable steps to ensure patient safety.)

Independent Contractors and Their Staffs

Another exception to vicarious liability concerns independent contractors, including contract agency healthcare providers and their employees. The legal system distinguishes employees, for whom an employer generally is legally responsible, from contractors, for whom an employer generally is not legally responsible. This distinction is based primarily on the degree of control the employer exercises over the physical details of the professional's work product.

In some cases, courts may hold employers vicariously liable even for contractors' actions under a legal theory called *apparent agency*. When a contract healthcare provider in a clinic is indistinguishable from an employee in the eyes of patients, for example, the law may treat the contract healthcare provider as an employee for purposes of vicarious liability. Therefore, prudent healthcare employers should take appropriate steps to ensure that patients know when they are being treated by contract professionals rather than by employees (e.g., by requiring contractors to wear name tags that identify their status as contract personnel, and/or by posting photographs identifying employees and contract professionals in a clinic reception area).

PRIMARY EMPLOYER LIABILITY FOR ACTIONS OF EMPLOYEES AND CONTRACTORS

A healthcare organization or system may be directly or primarily liable for employees' or contractors' conduct. Such liability exists independent of any vicarious liability that may also apply. An employer is directly liable under the legal concepts of negligent selection and retention, for example, for the wrongful actions of employees or contractors whom the employer reasonably should have: (1) rejected for employment, (2) carried out remediation for deficiencies for, or (3) discharged from employment.

Under law, hospitals and private clinics have certain responsibilities that they may not delegate to employees, professional medical staff, or independent contractors, under a legal concept called *corporate liability*. Such responsibilities are called *nondelegable duties*. Under corporate liability theories, courts have imposed various nondelegable duties on hospitals, including the following, among others: (1) a duty to use due care when selecting, privileging, and recredentialing physicians and surgeons and when evaluating the credentials and privileges (as applicable) of other primary healthcare providers; (2) a duty to ensure that premises and medical equipment are safe and adequate for patients, visitors, and staff; (3) a duty to establish patient care quality standards for their organizations and departments and divisions, and to monitor and evaluate the quality of patient care on an ongoing basis; and (4) a duty to continuously monitor the competence of professional and support personnel within the facility.

LIABILITY FOR PATIENT ABANDONMENT

Legally actionable abandonment of a patient occurs when a healthcare provider improperly unilaterally terminates a professional relationship with a patient and may be classified either as professional negligence or intentional misconduct, depending on the circumstances of the abandonment of the patient. Many patient care-related activities can constitute actionable abandonment, from momentarily leaving a patient unattended to refusing to work overtime during an emergency. Although a healthcare provider has almost absolute discretion in electing whether to form a professional relationship with a patient, certain legal rules must be complied with to terminate an existing patient–professional relationship properly. The law imposes a special duty of care on a healthcare provider caring for a patient, similar to the special duty owed by an attorney to a client or a parent or guardian to a child under his or her charge.

Patient abandonment has become a greater issue because of managed care, under which considerations of cost containment may cause third party payers to limit patient care to a set number of visits. Healthcare clinical professionals, not administrators or clerical personnel, are legally charged to determine the duration of patient care. Clinicians must take reasonable steps to appeal, when appropriate, administrative length-of-care decisions adverse to their patients and in contravention to their clinical judgment. Careful and appropriate documentation of justifications and rationale for such appeals (in patient health records and even in memoranda not filed in patient records) are crucial to generate and maintain in order to justify such appeals, and to minimize the likelihood of patient abandonment liability for clinical healthcare professionals.

Termination of the healthcare provider–patient relationship is justified when the patient makes a knowing, voluntary election to end the relationship, either unilaterally or jointly with the provider. The provider may initiate termination of the professional relationship with the patient when a medical condition under care has resolved. Unilateral termination of the relationship by the provider also properly may occur when, in a rehabilitation health professional's judgment, the patient has reached the zenith of his or her rehabilitative potential. Such a situation requires careful documentation in the patient's care record that will pass legal scrutiny should a healthcare malpractice action arise. (How to document such a situation and others discussed herein are addressed in later chapters.) Also, a healthcare professional must always communicate the fact that the patient has been discharged to a referring entity any time a patient has received care pursuant to a referral.

Negligent Abandonment

If a patient claims that he or she was discharged prematurely, then the legal action that results may be a professional negligence-based healthcare malpractice action. As with any other health professional negligence case, the plaintiff-patient will have to prove the following four elements by a preponderance, or the greater weight, of evidence: (1) the provider owed a duty of care to the patient; (2) the provider violated the duty by negligently unilaterally terminating the professional relationship prematurely; (3) the provider's improper discharge of the patient caused harm to the patient ("causation"); and (4) the patient suffered legally cognizable damages, such as pain and suffering, additional medical expenses, and lost wages that warrant the award of money damages to attempt to make the patient whole.

Intentional Abandonment

In contrast to negligent abandonment of a patient, a healthcare provider also may be charged with intentional abandonment of a patient, which carries with it more serious adverse consequences. As an intentional tort, intentional abandonment carries with it the possibility of a punitive (exemplary, i.e., "making an example") damages award should the patient prevail at trial. In most cases, the defendant's professional liability insurer will not be obligated (or even permitted) to indemnify the insured if the intentional conduct is adjudged to be sufficiently egregious to justify the imposition of punitive damages against the defendant-healthcare provider.

Intentional abandonment might involve situations in which a patient is discharged for reasons such as failure to pay a bill, a personality conflict with a treating healthcare professional, or an insurance denial of reimbursement for further care. Under such circumstances, the provider must, at a minimum, give advance notice to the patient of the provider's intent to terminate the relationship; give the patient a reasonable amount of time to find a suitable substitute healthcare provider, and assist the patient in finding a suitable substitute healthcare provider, if applicable. Any information about the patient—examination findings, diagnosis, or intervention-related data—must be communicated to the substitute care provider expeditiously. The provider transferring the patient must be sure to document in the patient's record the patient's health status at the time of discharge. As a risk-management measure, such a provider transferring a patient should also carefully memorialize in risk management documentation the steps undertaken to assist the patient in finding a substitute care provider. This can be done in the form of an office memorandum, which should be retained for the period of the statute of limitations and then only disposed of under advisement of the provider's or healthcare organization's legal counsel.

Substitute Healthcare Providers

Two special situations bear mentioning. One basis for an abandonment complaint might be that a healthcare provider left a patient in the care of a substitute healthcare provider while the original provider went on vacation, to a conference, or elsewhere for personal or business reasons. In settings in which patients contract for care with specific named clinicians, such as may occur in outpatient private practice settings, such providers must be sure to obtain and document the patients' informed consent before transferring care to substitute healthcare providers. (In hospital and health maintenance organization [HMO] settings, by contrast, patients do not normally contract for care with specific healthcare providers, so that the issue of abandonment during vacations and other periods of coverage does not normally arise involving providers in such settings.)

Abandonment Issues in the Limited Scope Practice Setting

Another problem concerns providers such as medical physicians, psychologists, social workers, physical and occupational therapists, nurse practitioners, dieticians, and other healthcare professionals who operate limited-scope practices. Consider as an example a nurse practitioner specializing exclusively in the care of pediatric and adolescent patients with orthopedic or sports-related injuries. Is such a provider at liberty to refuse to treat an unrelated condition involving a current patient? The answer is probably "yes"; however, the clinician must inform the patient before forming the health professional–patient relationship of the limited nature of his or her practice and obtain the patient's informed consent to undergo limited-scope care. Effective documentation of the patient's informed consent to limited-scope care can be crucial in avoiding health-care malpractice abandonment liability should a claim or lawsuit arise.

When a Healthcare Professional May Be Required to "Abandon" a Patient

Certain circumstances may require a treating healthcare professional to disengage from caring for a patient, such as when the provider termi-nates his or her employment with a hospital or clinic, or when a patient's third-party reimbursement for care terminates. Depending on the cir-cumstances in each particular case, such a provider may be required to continue necessary care on a *pro bono*, or free-of-charge basis, even when third-party reimbursement terminates. Providers and healthcare orga-nizations should always consult with their attorneys before discharging patients still in need of care under such circumstances.

BASES OF LIABILITY OTHER THAN NEGLIGENCE

The vast majority of reported healthcare malpractice legal cases involve allegations of professional negligence by providers. This is so in large part because courts are reluctant to allow patients to sue for non-negligence-based breach of contract in the healthcare setting, in part because of the special status relationship between primary healthcare professionals and patients. Similarly, courts hesitate to permit patients to sue healthcare pro-viders over injuries from defective products because the delivery of health care is generally viewed as the rendition of a professional service, not the sale of a product. This is changing, however, as more and more healthcare professionals market care-related products in their clinical practices in order to generate necessary revenue in the managed care practice envi-ronment. In such cases, courts may permit imposition of strict product liability when dangerous, defectively designed or manufactured healthcare products injure patients, their family members, and other third parties.

Few healthcare malpractice cases generally are premised exclusively on the issue of a lack of informed consent. Still, this blended ethical-legal area of responsibility is of great importance for all clinicians. Every primary healthcare provider is legally and ethically responsible for obtaining patients' informed consent before treatment. This important area of law and ethics is explored in greater detail in Chapter 4.

OTHER SETTINGS AND CONSEQUENCES OF MALPRACTICE ACTIONS

Criminal Proceedings for Conduct That Also Constitutes Malpractice

Besides a civil malpractice lawsuit, a health professional alleged to engage in gross (substantial) negligence, reckless conduct, or intentional misconduct may face criminal legal proceedings and adverse administrative actions before licensure boards and certification entities. Criminal actions are judicial proceedings but differ from civil malpractice legal actions in that a state or federal prosecutor brings the criminal case against the defendant on behalf of public interests, rather than the interests of an individual victim. Because the prospective penalties and stigma are more severe, the standard of proof—beyond a reasonable doubt—is much higher than the preponderance of evidence (or greater weight of evidence) standard generally in effect in civil court and administrative legal proceedings.

The consequences of a finding of liability in a civil malpractice trial and a finding of guilt in a criminal trial are also different. If a civil defendant is adjudged liable, the patient-plaintiff normally is awarded compensatory money damages for expenses such as lost wages, medical expenses, pain and suffering, loss of enjoyment of life, and property losses. Normally, a civil defendant's insurer indemnifies the insured and pays off such a money judgment. In egregious cases involving reckless or intentional misconduct, a civil jury or judge may award punitive damages to a plaintiff, for which a defendant's insurer might lawfully refuse to indemnify. The penalties for a criminal defendant found guilty of a crime normally are limited to incarceration (or the threat of incarceration, i.e., probation or confinement to one's home) and a monetary fine.

Administrative and Professional Affiliation Actions

Adverse administrative actions affecting license and/or certification affecting the very ability to practice one's profession may be taken by state administrative licensing agencies and certification entities, and, in the case of a health professional license, typically require a hearing to protect the constitutional due process rights of the respondent (the administrative equivalent of a "defendant"). Private professional association actions affecting professional association membership likewise may result from healthcare malpractice actions that involve professional ethical infractions.

MALPRACTICE TRIAL PRACTICE AND PROCEDURES

Roles of Healthcare Professionals in Malpractice Proceedings

A healthcare provider can take one of three roles in a civil malpractice proceeding: fact witness, expert witness, or defendant. The *fact witness* is probably the most familiar role. Also called an *eyewitness* or *percipient witness*, the fact witness possesses relevant firsthand knowledge about the issues and merits of a legal case important to one or both sides. A percipient witness might include a healthcare clinician or extender, an aide, or a chaperone who observed patient care activities involving a patient-litigant. Like experts and defendants, fact witnesses may be called upon to answer questions in interviews or under oath in depositions by one or both parties in a case during the pretrial, case-building "discovery" phase of the trial process. Fact witnesses normally do not have the discretion to withhold their testimony or admissible opinions, and they normally testify subject to a subpoena or court order. Fact witnesses are normally reimbursed according to fixed (low) statutory fee schedules, rather than being allowed the opportunity that expert witnesses have to negotiate higher fees with the party calling them to testify.

Primary nonphysician healthcare professionals find themselves more frequently in the role of healthcare malpractice defendant, as disciplines other than medicine are increasingly swept up in the malpractice litigation crisis. As a party defendant, a healthcare professional faces serious adverse professional and personal consequences should a verdict be rendered against him or her, including monetary losses, loss of reputation and goodwill, and adverse administrative actions at the state and federal levels. This fact is not presented with the intention to frighten healthcare providers into practicing and documenting patient care defensively. Rather, it is to familiarize them with the legal system and its processes, and to make them aware of the need to sequester patient care records and seek out and obtain legal representation expeditiously whenever a potentially compensable event such as a patient injury ripens into a claim or lawsuit. It is vitally important to follow legal counsel's advice and, in particular, to refrain from talking about any potential or actual legal action against you with anyone except counsel or counsel's agents (e.g., paralegal professionals and investigators working for the healthcare provider's attorney). The same admonition applies to written correspondence about a pending case when you are a healthcare malpractice defendant. Do not send any out, without legal counsel's review and concurrence!

Pretrial Proceedings

A healthcare provider must notify his or her facility legal department, personal professional liability insurance representative, and personal attorney immediately upon receipt of any legal papers concerning a patient's care. When a lawsuit is filed, the first papers served normally are the *summons* (notice of an impending lawsuit) and the *complaint* (specifying an incident or events allegedly causing a patient injury as well as the amount of money damages sought against the defendant-healthcare professional or organization). An insurer will expeditiously assign legal counsel to the case to file an *answer* to the patient-plaintiff 's initial *pleadings*.

Once the complaint, answer, and other responsive papers have been exchanged and filed with the court having *jurisdiction* (control) over the case, pretrial discovery begins in earnest. The parties to the lawsuit may require each other (but not each other's witnesses) to answer formal questions called *interrogatories*. The defendant-healthcare provider may even be called on by the plaintiff to concede liability in what is called a *request for admission*. Documents, including authenticated or certified copies of patient treatment records, will be requested by the patient's attorney, and other tangible evidence, such as equipment used in the course of treatment, may have to be produced for inspection by the plaintiff 's expert(s).

Depositions: Procedures and Precautions

The deposition is probably the most familiar discovery device, because many healthcare professionals have undergone depositions as expert witnesses or potential or actual malpractice defendants in the past. A deposition consists of sworn testimony of a party or potential party to a lawsuit, or of a fact or expert witness. It is usually taken in the office of the attorney representing the *deponent* (person being deposed) or in another seemingly informal neutral environment. To reduce stress, try to avoid being deposed at your place of work, such as a healthcare organization, where, among other things, interruptions by staff, patients, vendors, and others might affect your necessary concentration on the legal proceedings.

Irrespective of where a deposition takes place, do not as a deponent be lulled into a false sense of security because of the apparent informality of the deposition process. A deposition is a serious legal proceeding, the consequences of which are as important as trial testimony. A court reporter transcribes every word—formal and informal, "on" or "off" record—that every participant in the deposition says. The transcribed deposition may later be introduced at trial, especially to refute trial testimony that may be inconsistent with prior sworn testimony given at the deposition.

If healthcare professionals reading this section take just one piece of advice from it, it is that **they should never undergo a deposition either as a witness or defendant without prior consultation with and preparation by their attorneys**. This does not mean that every deponent needs to have an attorney present to represent him or her at deposition. Bear in mind, though, that a health professional-deponent called on to testify as a witness to an event may be named as a healthcare malpractice defendant the next day as a result of deposition testimony. One of the primary purposes of depositions is for attorneys for both plaintiff(s) and defendant(s) to discover relevant facts that will lead to evidence that will enable them to prevail at trial, or to facilitate a pretrial settlement of the case.

Healthcare Professionals as Expert Witnesses

The overwhelming majority of malpractice (and all other legal) cases are disposed of through means short of resorting to trial, principally through pretrial settlement or outright dismissal of cases. Should a healthcare malpractice case progress to trial, however, the verdict will probably turn on expert testimony. Healthcare professionals may qualify as experts for many purposes (e.g., as rehabilitation consultants regarding patient-plaintiffs' rehabilitation or vocational needs or potential). However, the principal area in which they testify as experts in malpractice proceedings is as clinical experts on whether a defendant-healthcare provider's treatment of a patient-plaintiff met or fell below (*breached*) the legal standard of care.

An expert witness on the standard of care may testify for either the patient-plaintiff or for the healthcare provider or organization-defendant. To meet the legal standard of care and avoid being adjudged negligent, a clinical healthcare professional caring for a patient must exercise that special knowledge and skill characteristic of reasonably competent peers acting under the same or similar circumstances. More specifically, a healthcare professional-defendant is expected by law to use examination, evaluative, diagnostic, prognostic, and intervention techniques and procedures that constitute at least minimally acceptable professional practice. Always bear in mind that legally acceptable care equates to minimally acceptable standards of practice, not necessarily what is optimal or even average. "Best care" is not at issue; the legal standard of care focuses on the "floor," not the "ceiling."

Before testifying as an expert on a professional standard of care, a witness must first be qualified as legally *competent*, based on expertise concerning the specific aspect of patient care at issue in the case. Oftentimes, the opponent's attorney will offer to stipulate to the qualifications of an expert witness. In such a case, the judge and jury do not have an opportunity to hear about the expert's academic background, professional publications history, or other individual attributes and achievements. Counsel presenting a witness as an expert may wish, in such situations, to seek the court's permission to enter the witness's qualifications into the record anyway. This exposure to the expert's qualifications will enhance the credibility of the expert in the eyes of the fact-finder and may lead to the fact-finder giving greater weight to the expert's testimony and opinions during deliberations on liability.

Erickson identified three cardinal attributes of an expert witness: (1) consistent superior performance, (2) successful practice outcomes, and (3) measurable, replicable processes and results. Liptak opined that experts selected by the parties instead of by the court are less helpful to juries in deciding cases. (In most other nations, judges appoint what are supposed to be only neutral experts in legal cases.)

A very important item of documentation in support of healthcare malpractice litigation is the expert witness report. This document is used by plaintiff-patients and defendant-healthcare providers and organizations to bolster their cases. Anyone serving as a consulting expert to a party to litigation should coordinate with the employing legal counsel before reducing an oral report to writing. Written expert witness reports may be legally "discoverable" by opposing counsel, even though they are considered semiprotected "attorney-work product." Ideas generated by an expert working for an attorney, however, enjoy greater protection from involuntary release than expert conclusions under a deliberative processes exemption.

All healthcare professionals should consider it a civic duty to honor a request by an attorney or a court or other public agency to testify as an expert on the standard of care in a case or administrative legal action. If health professionals from within the same discipline as a healthcare professional-defendant under charges do not come forward and assume responsibility for so testifying, members of other disciplines may fill the void and opine on another profession's practice standards, perhaps in an incomplete or incorrect manner. Attorneys and judges in individual cases will normally seek out appropriate expert witnesses from academic and clinical settings, or through referral by litigants and others in the trial process.

Potential and current expert witnesses must maintain and disseminate a fee schedule to prospective clients. The fee schedule for services must be reasonable for the market to be legal and ethical. Components of a fee schedule include charges for consulting, reviewing patient care records and other documents, report writing, travel time, and testifying either at deposition or at trial. Once an expert commits to being a testifying expert, he or she is ethically bound to live up to that commitment,

Some states have enacted tort reform legislation that affects expert witness reports. In Texas, for example, patient-plaintiffs in healthcare malpractice legal actions must serve an expert witness report (including the expert's curricula vitae) on each party within 120 days after filing a healthcare malpractice lawsuit. The expert report must include a summary of the expert's opinion on the legal standard of care; how it was breached by the defendant in the case; and how the defendant's breach of the standard of care caused injury to the patient-plaintiff. Failure to serve this summary expert opinion report automatically results in dismissal of a patient-plaintiff's case, with the added requirement to pay for the defendant's legal costs and attorney's fees. These measures help prevent frivolous legal actions from proceeding to depositions and trial, and unnecessarily clogging an already overcrowded legal system.

With tens of millions of civil lawsuits filed or pending in state and federal courts in the United States, far ahead of all other civilized nations combined, there clearly is a serious litigation crisis in the United States. In larger or relatively more litigious states, civil cases, including healthcare malpractice lawsuits, take many years to come to trial.

THE NATIONAL PRACTITIONER DATA BANK

Since September 1990, whenever money (in any sum) is paid to a patient-plaintiff or his or her representative, either in settlement or by way of a court judgment in a healthcare malpractice case, information about the responsible healthcare provider must be forwarded to the Department of Health and Human Services for inclusion in the National Practitioner Data Bank. This Data Bank was established pursuant to the Health Care Quality Improvement Act of 1986.

Another important purpose of the Data Bank is to compile data concerning adverse licensing, credentialing, and other actions, including expulsion from professional associations, involving licensed healthcare providers. Together, malpractice payment reporting and adverse actions reporting are intended to create a record designed to protect the patient-public that follows licensed healthcare professionals included in the Data Bank wherever in the United States they might seek employment.

Employers of licensed healthcare professionals are required under the statute to query the Data Bank regarding new employees and at regular intervals thereafter. The information is deemed strictly confidential and normally is not "discoverable" by patients or their attorneys, nor is it available to the general public. As an exception to the nondisclosure provision, if a healthcare employer fails to query the Data Bank about a provider upon employment, a patient-plaintiff's attorney may petition for, and be granted, access to that provider's Data Bank information. Any licensed healthcare provider may self-query the Data Bank for a nominal fee for his or her own record.

PATIENT CARE DOCUMENTATION AND TORT REFORM MEASURES

The federal government and most state legislatures have undertaken, since the advent of the litigation and healthcare malpractice crises, reforms focused on patient care documentation. Many of these public entities have also undertaken measures labeled as "tort reform" to decrease the number of civil lawsuits. One of these measures—expeditious filing of expert witness reports—has already been discussed. Some of the other tort reform measures include the following:

1. Enacting and, after substantial delay, implementing the Health Insurance Portability and Accountability Act (HIPAA) of 1996. This federal statute, focused on patients' protected health information (PHI), is discussed in detail in Chapter 6.

2. Limiting time periods for validity of undated patient health information release authorizations.

3. Requiring that healthcare malpractice plaintiffs undergo administrative hearings on the merits of their cases before proceeding to trial.

4. Capping maximum noneconomic money damages for pain and suffering and loss of enjoyment of life. (Note that this reform has been introduced on a yearly basis in Congress for over a decade without success. Bills introduced typically limit emotional pain and suffering damages to $250,000 as well as limiting attorney contingent fees. The nonpartisan Congressional Budget Office has predicted that such a federal tort reform law would reduce healthcare expenditures attributable to malpractice from 2 to 1.5 percent of aggregate medical costs.)

5. Limiting attorney contingent fees (contingent fees are based on percentages of recovery fees bargained for between attorneys and clients). California was the first state to do this in 1975.

6. Reforming "joint and several liability" to prevent one defendant from being required to pay an entire judgment when that defendant is only partially responsible for a plaintiff's injuries.

7. Setting absolute time limits—based on the date of manufacture of a product—within which legal action must be commenced (called *statutes of repose*).

8. Relaxing the "collateral source rule," under which juries are prevented from learning of a plaintiff's collateral sources of compensation for injuries, including insurance coverage or partial payments by other defendants.

9. Penalizing attorneys and their clients for initiating lawsuits deemed to be frivolous, especially in the federal courts.

10. Withholding from plaintiffs (and depositing in state treasuries) a percentage of any *punitive* (punishment) damages awarded to them by juries in product liability actions.

CHAPTER SUMMARY

All healthcare professionals, organizations, and systems are affected by the litigation and healthcare malpractice crises, characterized by increasing numbers and severity (cost) of claims and lawsuits, including those brought by patients claiming malpractice-related injuries. The overwhelming majority of healthcare malpractice cases are based on allegations of professional negligence, or substandard delivery of care. Whether a healthcare provider retrospectively met or violated minimally acceptable practice standards is normally determined through testimony of expert witnesses, or reference to relevant professional texts, peer-reviewed journals, and practice standards, guidelines, and protocols.

Employers of healthcare providers may be vicariously or indirectly liable for employees', volunteers', and even independent contractors' commission of healthcare malpractice. Healthcare organizations may also be independently liable for violating nondelegable duties owed to patients and others, including the duty to select and retain only competent healthcare professionals, the duty to maintain safe premises and equipment, and the duty to oversee the quality of patient care provided in their facilities. Clinical managers and practitioners also need to carefully establish procedures delineating the circumstances under which healthcare providers may disengage from further care of patients to minimize allegations of negligent or intentional patient abandonment. This issue is particularly important under the current cost containment-focused managed care paradigm.

Healthcare providers must expeditiously notify their facility risk managers, insurers, and personal legal representatives whenever an incident occurs in the clinic that might conceivably ripen into a claim or lawsuit. Such occurrences are called potentially compensable events. A claim of healthcare malpractice ripens into formal legal civil proceedings when a defendant-healthcare provider receives a summons and complaint specifying the basis of the alleged malpractice and a demand for money damages or other relief.

One of the most important pretrial proceedings is the deposition, in which parties and witnesses to malpractice lawsuits undergo examination under oath by the parties' attorneys. Never go into a deposition, either as a witness or defendant, without prior consultation and preparation by legal counsel. The deposition serves several important functions, including locking in sworn testimony weeks, months, or years before trial and discovering facts that might lead to additional relevant evidence in the case.

The consequences of healthcare malpractice legal actions are potentially devastating for both patients affected by substandard care and healthcare professionals whose reputations and personal well-being are affected by such allegations, whether or not the allegations are substantiated as true. Licensed healthcare professionals on whose behalf malpractice judgments or settlements are paid face the additional penalty of having their names included in the National Practitioner Data Bank, maintained by the federal Department of Health and Human Services. For these reasons, and for the protection of patients and healthcare professionals alike, management of healthcare malpractice risk in clinical practice, particularly through creating and maintaining accurate, complete, objective, and timely documentation of patient care activities, is critically important.

The United States is the most litigious nation on earth and in world history. In an effort to stem the numbers of civil lawsuits initiated in state and federal courts, courts and legislatures are taking ongoing actions to dampen the malpractice fervor through procedural and substantive restrictions on plaintiffs' ability to bring civil tort lawsuits. Such measures collectively are called tort reform. Resort to alternative dispute resolution—mediation and arbitration—is an effective and cost-saving means of reducing the number of formal civil lawsuits in the long pipeline.

REFERENCES AND SUGGESTED READINGS

American Health Lawyers Association. Washington, D.C. Homepage. Accessed June 11, 2011, from http://www.healthlawyers.org

Eickhoff J. Exercise equipment injuries: Who's at fault? *ACSM's Health & Fitness Journal.* 2002; 6(1):27–30.

Erickson KA. The making of an expert. *Harvard Business Review.* 2007; 85(8): 115–121.

Furrow B, Greaney T, Johnson S, Jost T, Schwartz R. *Health Law: Cases, Materials and Problems*, 6th ed. St. Paul, MN: Thomson-West Publishing Co; 2008.

The Great Medical Malpractice Hoax: NPBDB Data Continue to Show Medical Liability System Produces Rational Outcomes. Washington, DC: Public Citizen Congress Watch; 2007. Accessed June 11, 2011, from http://www.citizen.org/publications/publicationredirect.cfm?ID=7497

Greater Southeast Community Hosp. Found. v. Walker, 313 A.2d 105 (D.C. 1973).

Guide to Physical Therapist Practice, 2nd ed. rev. Alexandria, VA: American Physical Therapy Association; 2004.

Hanks GC, Polinger-Hymen R. Redefining the battlefield: Expert reports in medical malpractice litigation after HB4. *Texas Bar Journal.* 2004; December:936–944.

HealthGrades. Denver, CO. Homepage. Accessed June 11, 2011, from http://www.healthgrades.com

Institute of Medicine of the National Academies. Washington, D.C. Homepage. Accessed June 11, 2011, from http://www.iom.edu

Kearney KA, McCord FL. Hospital management faces new liabilities. *Health Law.* 1992; Fall:1–6.

Keeton WP. *Prosser and Keeton on Torts*, 5th ed. St. Paul, MN: West Law Publishers, Inc; 1984.

Leape LL, Berwick DM. Five years after "To Err Is Human," what have we learned? *JAMA.* 2005; 293:2384–2390.

Leitner DL. *Managed Care Liability.* Chicago: American Bar Association (Tort and Insurance Practice Section); 1996.

Liptak A. Experts hired to shed light can leave US courts in dark. *New York Times.* August 12, 2008:A1, 16.

Lopopolo RB, Schafer DS, Nosse LJ. Leadership, administration, management, and professionalism (LAMP) in physical therapy: a Delphi Study. *Physical Ther.* 2004; 84(2):137–150.

Myer v. Woodall, 592 P.2d 1343 (Colo. Ct. App. 1979).

National Practitioner Data Bank, Department of Health and Human Services, Chantilly, VA. Homepage. Accessed June 11, 2011, from http://www.npdb-hipdb.hrsa.gov

Novey v. Kishawaukee Community Health Serv., 531 N.E.2d 427 (Ill. App. Cf. 4989).

Physical Therapy Claims Study. Chicago: CNA HealthPro; 2006.

Rosenbaum DE. Debate on malpractice looms for senate. *New York Times.* December 20, 2004:A16.

Scott RW. *Promoting Legal and Ethical Awareness: A Primer for Health Professionals and Patients*. St. Louis, MO: Mosby-Elsevier, Inc; 2009.

Texas Civil Practice and Remedies Code Annotated, Section 74.351 (Vernon 2005 & Supp. 2006).

REVIEW CASE STUDIES

The following case examples involve hypothetical situations and are not based on actual healthcare malpractice cases, published or unpublished. The characters are fictitious and are not intended to represent or resemble any actual healthcare provider or entity. Any resemblance of any examples in this text to actual cases, situations, individuals, or entities is coincidental and unintended.

1. A is an orthopedic patient with chronic cervical pain, being seen for the first time by B, an outpatient physical therapist. No documentation except the prescription, properly signed by the referring physician, is present with the patient at the initial visit. During the course of examination, B asks A if any x-rays had been taken. A replies "yes," and adds, "I think the doctor said they were OK." Should B proceed with mechanical traction treatment based on the examination findings and A's self-report about her x-rays?

2. X, a hand-care patient of Y, an occupational therapist, admits to Y that he is feigning a work-related hand injury in order to maximize compensation from the workers' compensation system. What documentation steps should Y take?

DISCUSSION: REVIEW CASE STUDIES

1. B probably should not proceed with A's mechanical cervical traction treatment without first reviewing the x-ray report or consulting with A's physician. A might have pathology that could make traction contraindicated. This is a common problem in clinical practice that can readily be resolved through communication between the referring entity and the treating provider, and through

conversion by healthcare providers and organizations to universally available electronic medical records (EMRs).

2. Y probably does not have a legal privilege to withhold, and may have a legal duty to disclose, X's workers' compensation fraud to authorities. Y should initially document the circumstances of X's disclosure in an incident report and seek immediate further guidance from her supervisor and legal counsel.

For the Suggested Answer Framework to the Focus on Ethics, please refer to Appendix D.

CHAPTER 2

Clinical Patient Care Documentation Methods and Management

This chapter overviews the nature and processes of clinical patient care documentation. The main purposes of healthcare documentation are discussed, with emphasis on the principal purpose for documenting: communication of vital health-related information about patients to other healthcare professionals having an imminent need to know. The chapter also explores the three principal formats for patient care record notation, and the essential contents of patient treatment records required to meet the legal standard of care. The chapter includes a Focus on Ethics vignette and concludes with discussion of 25 select documentation problems, errors, and suggestions, including case examples.

INTRODUCTION

No business activity in the United States, except for national defense, is as critically important to the welfare of the citizenry, or as costly, as the delivery of health care. Literally tens of millions of inpatient and outpatient visits—many with life and death consequences for patients—are logged annually throughout the United States. Annual health-related expenditures in the United States for 2010 totaled more than $2.6 trillion, and are estimated by the Census Bureau to be $4.3 trillion by 2018.

A substantial proportion of these costs are earmarked for administration, including for patient care documentation. The three areas of highest patient care documentation cost outlay are HIPAA compliance, reimbursement management activities, and conversion to electronic medical records. No business endeavor, including national defense, routinely requires the comprehensive and accurate documentation of client (patient) services (history, examination, evaluation, diagnosis, prognosis, and intervention) to the degree that the healthcare delivery system does.

As part of the legal duty owed to patients, every primary healthcare provider is required by legal, professional, and business ethical standards to record clinically pertinent history, examination, evaluative, and intervention-related information about their patients and to maintain that information in the form of patient treatment records. Besides primary healthcare providers (i.e., those licensed independent practitioners who can legally interact with patients without the requirement of a prior examination and referral by another healthcare provider), other healthcare professionals interacting with patients in supportive or consultative roles have the same duty to record patient information (if they are privileged under law and by their organizations to document) and ensure that it is safeguarded.

It is a truism that patient care documentation must be patient-focused. Providers must use people-first, active-voice language when describing patients, both orally and in writing. Mrs. Jones, for example, is "a 52-year-old woman presenting with right cerebral vascular accident (CVA)," not "a hemi."

Who can legally document information in patient records is a matter of federal and state law, organizational or systems policy, and customary practice. For inpatient records, therapeutic orders are normally written by medical physicians and surgeons attending individual patients. In most cases, no one except a physician can record information in the "Physician's Orders" section of an inpatient record, except where so permitted by law and custom, such as when a dental surgeon writes relevant orders for care for a specific patient. In outpatient patient care settings, however, especially in clinical settings in which no physician may be present, intervention orders are routinely written by primary healthcare providers other than physicians, for example, by nurse practitioners and by physical therapists in direct access or practice-without-referral jurisdictions.

Patient care records take many forms. Two primary classifications of patient care records include inpatient records and ambulatory, or outpatient, records. (Some authorities consider emergency treatment records as a separate third category of patient care records.) Although in the past, original patient treatment records were required by law to be handwritten in all jurisdictions, modernly, both inpatient and ambulatory records may be created originally and maintained, either in whole or in part, on a computer in most states. Electronic patient care documentation and conversion to electronic medical records is discussed in greater detail in Chapter 6.

It is difficult to enunciate a precise definition for a patient care record. In simplest terms, a patient care record is a memorialization of a specific patient's health status at a given point in time and over an extended time period. The patient treatment record includes clinically pertinent information that is clear, concise, comprehensive, individualized, accurate, objective, and timely. It serves both as a business document and as the legal record of care rendered to the patient.

From business and clinical perspectives as well as from a legal standpoint, documentation of patient care is as important as the rendition of care itself. This axiom holds true for the protection of patients and healthcare professionals alike. For healthcare providers, patient care documentation is substantive evidence of the nature, extent, and quality of care rendered to patients, whereas for patients, it serves as a permanent record of their health status, which may, among many other purposes, serve as a historical record for future lifesaving intervention.

> Documentation of patient care is as important as the rendition of care itself.

PURPOSES OF PATIENT CARE DOCUMENTATION

The patient care record serves a myriad of important purposes. Primary healthcare professionals and healthcare organizations act as fiduciaries, or persons and entities in a special position of trust vis-a-vis patients under their care. Therefore, logically, the primary purpose of patient care documentation is to communicate vital information about a patient's health status to other healthcare providers concurrently caring for that patient and having an imminent need to know the information contained therein. This principle operates in both inpatient and outpatient care settings. The clinical information entered by one healthcare professional in a patient's record is assimilated by other providers into their intervention plans, and incorporated with their goals for patients, to ease discomfort, speed recovery, and maximize function and independence.

Despite what may be suspected by some to be the primary purpose for patient care documentation—self-protection from patient-initiated claims and litigation—this is clearly not the case. That kind of negative approach to documentation serves no positive purpose and only instills fear in healthcare professionals. Such fear, in turn, fosters an atmosphere of costly overly defensive healthcare practice.

A blatant self-defensive presentation by a healthcare professional— especially regarding patient care documentation—may actually increase malpractice exposure. Patients and their significant others can often sense a healthcare provider's defensiveness. They justifiably find distasteful the kind of formal, cold, businesslike relationship that inherently results when a healthcare professional puts fear of malpractice exposure (or other self-interest, such as revenue maximization) ahead of the patient's welfare. If patients come to believe that their healthcare providers are excessively focused on self-protection from litigation exposure or other self-centered considerations, then they may be more inclined to pursue legal actions if and when an adverse outcome results from intervention.

There are many other important, recognized purposes of patient care documentation. Documentation of patient care serves as a basis for planning and for ensuring continuity of care in the future for patients currently under care, particularly for those inpatients who, after discharge, will require health professional intervention at home. By memorializing a patient's health status at any given point, documentation also serves to create a historical record of a given patient's health, from which data can be extracted for, and utilized in, future contingencies, ranging from emergent life-threatening crises to disability determinations.

Documentation also forms the basis for monitoring and assessing the quality of care rendered to patients as part of a quality management program. Such programs are required of healthcare facilities accredited by entities such as the Joint Commission (JC), the Commission on Accreditation of Rehabilitation Facilities (CARF), the National Committee on Quality Assurance (NCQA), and others, including local, state, and federal public oversight entities. JC, CARF, and NCQA are further discussed in Chapter 5.

Besides its utility as a database for monitoring and evaluating the quality of patient care, patient care documentation is useful as a productivity measure of provider workloads, and to assess whether healthcare providers are practicing effective utilization management of human and nonhuman healthcare resources. It also serves, through identifying deficiencies, to ascertain whether there are needs for training for healthcare providers, from communication skills to substantive aspects of patient care.

As a business document, the patient care record is also evaluated by governmental third-party payer entities such as Medicare, Medicaid, TriCare (for military beneficiaries), state and local governmental entities, and by insurance companies and other third-party payers to determine levels of reimbursement for patient care. Documentation of patient care, then, is the primary means of justifying reimbursement for treatment. Patient treatment records also provides information that is useful for scientific and clinical research and for education.

Besides being a business document, the patient care record is a legal document. In the event of a healthcare malpractice claim or lawsuit, providers' documentation of patient care activities provides substantive and relatively objective evidence of the care that was rendered to the patient claiming malpractice. Documented evidence of care recorded in the patient's record provides expert witnesses with a basis from which to form a professional opinion on whether a provider or multiple providers met or violated standards of practice and legal standards of care. Patient care documentation serves many other legal functions, too, including, among others, its use as substantive evidence of work or functional capacity in worker's compensation and similar administrative proceedings.

As an additional legal issue, documentation of patient-informed consent protects patients, providers, and healthcare organizations and systems by serving as written evidence that a patient actually understood the risks and benefits of specific interventions and made a knowing, informed choice to undergo examination and accept recommended interventions. Documentation of a patient's desires in the event of that patient's mental incapacitation through advance directives serves also to memorialize patient decisions, evidence respect for patient autonomy, and protect healthcare professionals who must carry out the patient's valid advance directives.

Purposes of Patient Care Documentation

1. Communicates vital information about a patient's health status to other healthcare providers concurrently caring for that patient and having an immediate need to know the information contained therein

2. Acts as a basis for patient care planning and continuity of care

3. Serves as the primary source of information for assessing the quality of patient care rendered

4. Provides information for reimbursement and utilization review decisions

5. Identifies provider deficiencies and training needs

6. Serves as a resource for research and education

7. Serves as a business document

8. Serves as a multipurpose legal document

9. Provides substantive evidence on whether providers' care rendered, and healthcare organizations' oversight of patient care activities, met or violated legal standards of care

10. Memorializes through advance directives patient informed consent to examination and intervention as well as patient desires regarding life-sustaining measures in the event of a patient's subsequent mental incapacitation

CONTENTS OF PATIENT CARE RECORDS

Required contents of patient care records vary greatly depending on, among other considerations, state and federal laws and regulations, accreditation standards, organization and system requirements, and patient care settings. For hospitalized patients, for example, patient records are typically divided into two parts: (1) intake, or admissions data, including the relevant patient histories and assessments, physical examinations by admitting physicians (including admission studies and tests) and other primary healthcare professionals, and the admission diagnosis or diagnoses; and (2) the clinical record, in which progress notes, consultations, laboratory tests, diagnostic imaging studies, operative and anesthesia reports, and discharge summaries are written. Contents of outpatient records display greater variation.

FORMATS FOR PATIENT CARE DOCUMENTATION

Because communication of patient information to other healthcare professionals concurrently caring for that patient is of such critical importance, clinicians must ensure that their documentation of a patient's health status is understood by others on the healthcare team. This section discusses acceptable formats for communicating patient information to others. Practical considerations for effective documentation are considered in the next section.

Practically, there are only three general patient care documentation formats, whether handwritten or in electronic documentation format: narrative format, template (or report) format, and acronym/initialism format. The simplest form of patient care documentation is in narrative, or free-form, format. The prose form of literary composition, used by students in papers, theses, and dissertations, is the most common example of narrative format. Template or report format utilizes word and phrase prompts and blank spaces to generate and record data. Electronic documentation systems commonly utilize the template format. The acronym/initialism format employs alphabetic letters to form words (acronyms) or initialize data. "SOAP" (subjective-objective-assessment-plan) is an example of the acronym format; "PSP" (problem-status-plan) is an example of initialism format. The three basic patient care documentation formats may be combined into hybrid formats, and all three are equally amenable to being accessed by computer.

The acronym SOAP was originally developed by Dr. Lawrence Weed at the University of Vermont in the late 1960s to standardize physician, nursing, and physical and occupational therapy patient care documentation. It is part of the highly structured problem-oriented medical record system (POMR).

Each of these three formats offers relative advantages and disadvantages. The principal advantages of the narrative format are that it is the most flexible of formats and does not limit the amount of data that writers can annotate. Its disadvantages are that it does not compartmentalize information into readily discernible categories and that it facilitates verbosity by writers. The template or report format's key advantages are that information is neatly compartmentalized and standardization maximized through its use. Its disadvantages include that it may facilitate underdocumentation (e.g., when all blank spaces are not addressed) and that special circumstances may be difficult to address, or may be relegated to a miscellaneous section on the form. Acronym/initialism formats share the compartmentalization advantage that characterizes the template or report format. SOAP format (discussed in greater detail later) is so universally utilized by healthcare providers and organizations that its use may facilitate faster processing of information by users and thus enhance communication.

The problem-oriented SOAP approach highlights key information, including historical information about a patient and his or her chief complaint, clinical examination findings and objective observations of the examining clinician, the diagnosis (or diagnoses) or evaluative findings, and a proposed plan of intervention for the patient. In essence, both acronym/initialism and template/report formats are problem-oriented. Narrative patient care documentation, on the other hand, often makes critical patient information difficult to locate expeditiously.

More on SOAP

In SOAP format, patient information is compartmentalized into four main sections of an initial note: the subjective element ("S"), the objective element ("O"), the assessment ("A"), and the plan ("P"). Collectively, these elements compose the problem-oriented SOAP note documentation model. Under the SOAP note format, healthcare professionals can quickly access pertinent information recorded by another provider who conducted a prior examination of a patient by referring to the four elements of the SOAP note.

The "S," or subjective, element of an initial SOAP note customarily includes the following information:

1. A patient's medical diagnosis (or diagnoses)

2. A summary of the patient's relevant health history taken from the patient interview and from a review of the patient's available records

3. The patient's expression of his or her condition, including parameters of symptoms, such as the location, quality (sharp, dull, throbbing), severity (minimal, moderate, severe along a visual analog scale), nature (constant, intermittent), and factors that increase or decrease pain; the presence or absence of sensory symptoms (e.g., paresthesia, anesthesia, and loss of normal proprioception [perception of joint position in space]); ambulation, balance, and coordination status; level of independence; and mental status

4. The patient's medication list, subjective reactions to medications being taken, and any allergies—documented or reported

Some clinicians create a separate section for the patient history and do not include it under the "S" element of a SOAP note.

Many patients provide a medication list, which becomes part of the examination documentation. Providers usually write "See attached list," rather than taking the time to write out all patient medications. Providers are cautioned to carefully monitor patients' medication lists, especially for medications that providers know or should have known have been withdrawn from the market, such as cyclooxygenase-2 (COX-2) inhibitors like Vioxx in November 2004. Electronic medical records, including computerized medication lists, routinely provide safeguards against unintended prescriptions and the concomitant use by patients of redundant or dangerous medications.

The "O" element of an initial SOAP note includes objective examination data and findings about the patient. These data might include skin appearance and tone; muscle, neurological, postural, and sensory examination results; the patient's activities of daily living (ADL) status; results of a gait analysis; analytical skills test results; reflex test findings; and laboratory test and diagnostic imaging report results.

The "A" element of an initial SOAP note represents the evaluating healthcare professional's clinical assessment, based on objective examination findings and subjective input from the patient and others, and on available patient health records.

The "P" element of an initial SOAP note delineates the primary clinician's intended plan of intervention for the patient. In this section, the clinician might also document that the patient gave informed consent to the examination and recommended intervention. If, in addition to being examined, the patient receives initial treatment, medication administration, or other intervention, then the objective and subjective results of such intervention should also be summarized under the "P" element of the initial note.

A fifth alphabetical initial may be added to the traditional SOAP format, that being a "G" for interventional goals. As outcome criteria, functional goals represent expectations of and for a patient regarding the patient's ability to carry out important ADLs. These goals are often subdivided into short-term goals (often abbreviated STG) and long-term goals (LTG).

Do Stated Treatment Goals Equate to a Legally Binding "Therapeutic Promise"?

A legal issue that sometimes arises in healthcare malpractice proceedings is whether patient goals established by a clinician in a patient care note represent a guarantee, or warranty, of a specific therapeutic result, for which the failure to achieve the goal may be labeled a breach of a therapeutic promise, resulting in contract-based liability on the part of the provider and/or healthcare organization. The answer to this question is generally no. Patient intervention goals are not promises made to a patient but, rather, are the written manifestation of the primary healthcare provider's professional clinical judgment. As such, goals merely represent the provider's professional opinion about expected outcomes of intervention. Healthcare providers are cautioned, however, that the actual communication of specific therapeutic promises to patients may very well create a binding legal obligation to meet the promises made, or to face liability for breach of contract if they are not achieved.

Summary of SOAPG Initial Patient Care Notation Format

S: Contains medical, medication, occupational, familial, and social historical information relevant to a specific patient's health condition or complaint, related by the patient to the primary healthcare professional or extracted from the patient's health record

O: Contains the results of examination findings, including relevant laboratory and diagnostic imaging results

A: Contains the primary clinician's evaluative assessment and clinical diagnosis/diagnoses

P: Contains the proposed plan of intervention for the patient, and may include documentation of the patient's informed consent to examination and intervention and receipt of HIPAA information. If initial intervention ensues, then a summary of results of initial care is also recorded

G: Contains short- and long-term functional goals (patient-generated expected functional outcomes) of intervention

Problem-Status-Plan (PSP) Initialism Format

A variation of the SOAP problem-oriented patient care documentation format often used for recording patient progress notes is the problem-status-plan (PSP) format. Under this format, a re-evaluation note will include the patient's problem(s) and prior evaluative findings and diagnosis (or diagnoses) under "P," the patient's subjective expression of his or her condition after treatment and the objective findings of the re-examination are listed under "S," and the revised plan of intervention is listed under the second "P." As with the SOAP format, some clinicians prefer to add a "G" element to this format as well, to memorialize their revised outcome criteria, or functional goals, based on the patient's ADL and work-related needs and desires.

Problem-Status-Plan (PSP) Documentation Format for Patient Re-evaluations

P: Contains a summary of the patient's prior evaluative findings and diagnosis (or diagnoses)

S: Contains subjective and objective information about the patient's condition upon reexamination

P: Contains the modified patient intervention plan, based on the current clinical findings

Examples of the formats discussed in this section appear in Appendix 2-A at the end of this chapter.

The examples of standardized documentation formats presented in this chapter represent only some of the many formats in use by primary and support healthcare providers, individually and collectively. No one format is *the* correct format for meeting the required legal standard of care for patient care documentation, or for ethically meeting the fiduciary duty owed to patients under care. As long as a particular format used by healthcare professionals working in concert promotes effective communication about their patients' health and conditions, then the format is legally acceptable and within the legal standard of care.

Considerations of third-party payer documentation requirements for reimbursement, although not a healthcare malpractice legal issue per se, are critically important, too, for the financial viability of healthcare professionals, organizations, and systems. Current and developing electronic medical records documentation formats facilitate the simultaneous compliance with regulatory (particularly HIPAA) and procedural documentation requirements of multiple third-party payers, and are highly recommended for use by providers and facilities.

Forms submitted to the Center for Medicare Services (CMS) by outpatient rehabilitation providers for reimbursement for eligible patient care (Forms 700 [Plan of Treatment], 701 [Updated Plan of Progress]), or equivalents, combine features of narrative, SOAP, and template formats. These forms include the following required information: patient/provider(s) administrative information and signatures certifying the necessity for care; patient problems and treatment diagnoses, summary of evaluation and findings; short-term, long-term, and patient goals; and the treatment plan.

RISK MANAGEMENT CONSIDERATIONS FOR EFFECTIVE PATIENT CARE DOCUMENTATION

Patient Care Documentation: The First Draft Is the Final Work Product

Imagine that you are an author of fiction novels. Several hours after signing a "contingent" book contract based on an outline proposal, your prospective publisher calls you on the telephone and demands that you begin writing immediately and submit a final product within one week. As an added burden, imagine that the publisher tells you that you will be allowed to submit only one draft of your novel, upon which a firm publication decision will be based. Impossible? Ludicrous?

Now imagine that you are a healthcare provider working in the emergency department of a regional trauma center. A critically injured patient is transported to your facility without notice. While other members of the team begin to examine the comatose patient, you begin to record the patient's vital signs on an admission form. The patient suddenly goes into cardiac arrest, and cardiopulmonary resuscitation immediately ensues. With all of the tension and haste inherent in this situation, your recording of the information shouted to you by surgeons and nurses reflects your state of nervousness. The entries are scribbled, and words, syllables, and rough diagrams take the place of full sentences and careful illustrations that otherwise would be standard procedure.

Now imagine that the patient's condition deteriorates, and she dies while in the emergency department. A healthcare malpractice lawsuit is filed, and it proceeds to trial. The attorney for the patient's estate and her survivors offers the emergency room admission record into evidence. The conduct of the medical team will probably be judged in large part on the basis of that record of care that, of necessity, was written in an atmosphere of haste and tension, without any opportunity for drafts or revisions. Similar circumstances occur in emergency departments, operating suites, and other locations throughout healthcare organizations literally tens of thousands of times each day.

Although not every patient care encounter demands that documentation of care be conducted "under the gun," in almost every situation healthcare clinical professionals interacting with patients are prohibited from revising or refining their initial examination or intervention patient care entries, because to do so would constitute *spoliation*, or the intentional destruction or alteration of patient care documents with the specific intent to hide or change their clear meaning. The conduct of healthcare providers, unlike with most other professionals, is routinely evaluated and judged on the basis of a first "draft" of their work product, that is, the patient care record.

PATIENT CARE DOCUMENTATION PROBLEMS, ERRORS, AND SUGGESTIONS

Because the consequences of patient care documentation entries are so critically important to effective management of healthcare malpractice risk exposure, this section presents 25 common patient care documentation problems, errors, and suggestions designed to minimize the incidence and effects of incomplete or legally substandard documentation. These scenarios are equally applicable to written and electronic patient care documentation formats. Some of the problems identified herein may seem so trivial and their solutions so obvious that they do not merit mentioning; however, very often in healthcare malpractice proceedings, the simplest, seemingly trite documentation mistakes have the most serious adverse impact on legal case outcomes. No one should think that his or her intelligence is being insulted by some of these apparently simplistic guidelines for patient care documentation; because the recommendations presented may help to prevent a finding of liability for healthcare malpractice and all its adverse consequences.

Twenty-Five Documentation Problems, Errors, and Suggestions

1. Documentation problem: Illegible notation

2. Documentation error: Failure to identify (or correctly identify) the patient under care

3. Documentation error: Failure to annotate the date (and time, depending on customary practice) of patient care activities

4. Documentation problem: Use of multiple or inconsistent documentation formats by providers in a facility

5. Documentation error: Failure to use an indelible instrument to record examination, evaluation, diagnostic, prognostic, intervention, or outcome data about a patient under care

6. Documentation problem: Pen runs out of ink midway through a patient care record entry

7. Documentation problem: Line spacing in patient care record entries

8. Documentation problem: Signing patient care record entries

9. Documentation problem: Error correction

10. Documentation error: Unauthorized and unrecognized abbreviations

11. Documentation errors: Improper spelling, grammar, and the use of extraneous verbiage not affecting patient care

12. Documentation problems: Transcription problems with physician orders; examining and intervening on behalf of patients without written orders, where legally required

13. Documentation error: Untimely documentation of patient care activities

14. Documentation error: Identifying or filing an incident report in the patient care record

15. Documentation problem: Failing to delineate patient care rendered or identify clinical information supplied by another provider

16. Documentation error: Blaming or disparaging another provider in the patient care record

17. Documentation error: Expressing personal feelings about a patient or patient family member or significant other in the patient care record

18. Documentation suggestion: Document observations and findings objectively

19. Documentation suggestion: Document with specificity

20. Documentation error: Recording "hearsay" (secondhand input) as fact

21. Documentation suggestion: Exercise special caution when countersigning another provider's, student's, or intern's patient care notation

22. Documentation error: Failure to document a patient's informed consent to examination and intervention

23. Documentation suggestion: Document thoroughly patient/family/significant other's understanding of, and safe compliance with, discharge, home care, and follow-up instructions

24. Documentation suggestion: Carefully document a patient's noncompliance with provider directives or recommendations

25. Documentation suggestion: Carefully document a patient's or family member/significant other's possible contributory negligence related to alleged patient injuries or lack of progress.

Documentation Problem: Illegible Notation

If there is one comment that patients make most often, it is probably that their physicians and other healthcare providers do not write legibly in patient health records. It might not surprise you to hear that healthcare professionals themselves also often cannot decipher one another's patient care record entries, causing them either to have to consult with the writer of an entry for "translation" or, worse yet, to disregard the illegible information or even an entire entry.

Electronic medical records, where in use, have dampened the overall severity of this problem somewhat. With electronic medical records, there is greater flexibility for healthcare clinicians, in that data are not normally saved as final until done so by the clinician writing the note or entry.

Even in emergency situations, there is no excuse for documenting patient care illegibly. Keep in mind that the primary purpose of patient care documentation is to communicate vital information about a patient to other healthcare professionals concurrently caring for that patient, and having an imminent need to know.

How many times have you had to struggle to try to decipher another healthcare provider's handwriting on an intervention order, in a consultation report, or in another document? Have you ever had to spend time trying to decipher your own prior patient care entries? Assuming that the latter situation has occurred on at least one occasion for all of us, imagine how embarrassing it would be to be asked by a patient's attorney during a deposition to read one of your own garbled notation entries, and not be able to do so. Or worse yet, to be asked to read it aloud before a judge, a jury, and 40 to 50 spectators at trial. The devastating effect that such a situation would have on a healthcare malpractice defendant-healthcare provider's or organization's case is self-evident.

Clinical managers and healthcare organization and system administrators must take whatever administrative steps are necessary to ensure that healthcare professionals within their domains of supervision and control write legibly. This may entail developing alternative documentation systems not based on handwritten notation for providers who cannot be made compliant. For example, the use of dictation and transcription of entries is a viable alternative to handwritten documentation for such primary healthcare professionals. Conversion to, and use of, electronic medical records can also alleviate the problem of illegible patient care documentation. When these systems are unavailable, individual providers who cannot write or print legibly should type or otherwise key in electronically their patient care entries. As a last (and drastic) resort, the retention of clinical privileges in a facility can and should be conditioned on the ability to communicate legibly with other providers and support personnel.

Providers themselves should also self-police to ensure that their handwritten patient care documentation is legible and neat. When necessary, print or type entries instead of writing in cursive. Remember that a negligent failure to communicate vital patient care information is itself a form of professional negligence-based healthcare malpractice and a legitimate basis for primary (direct) liability for resultant patient injury.

When a healthcare provider's illegible documentation of patient care information is the proximate cause of delayed treatment or patient injury, the failure to communicate effectively constitutes actionable healthcare malpractice.

Documentation Error: Failure to Identify (or Correctly Identify) the Patient Under Care

Failure to identify, or correctly identify, a patient under care in documentation is another form of negligence that can lead to malpractice liability. Every page of a patient's paper or electronic medical record must contain the patient's full name written in indelible ink or imprint, or in the form of a stamp. Each page should also contain appropriate personal identifying information about the patient to facilitate expedient communication with the patient or relevant others.

As a primary healthcare provider or supportive professional writing patient information on a document, you bear primary ethical and legal responsibility for ensuring that the patient written about is correctly identified on the document. As a matter of customary practice, do not relinquish control over a piece of paper involving patient care that you have written an entry on unless the patient's name and identifying information is on it.

Documentation Error: Failure to Annotate the Date (and Time, Depending on Customary Practice) of Patient Care Activities

Failure to annotate the date (and, where required, the time) of patient care can be a supporting factor in the imposition of healthcare malpractice liability. Accounting for the chronology of patient care is especially crucial for physicians and nurses administering medications to patients when a duplicate dose of the medication in issue might be toxic to the patient. Providers such as physical and occupational therapists, whose practice and utilization management standards set limits for the number of permissible interventions in a given time period, must also carefully annotate the dates (and perhaps times) of interventional activities. Date entries must always include the day, month, and year. To avoid confusion over AM and PM where treatment times are annotated, consider adopting the systematic use of military time (e.g., 0001 to 2400 hours).

Documentation Problem: Use of Multiple or Inconsistent Documentation Formats by Providers in a Facility

Effective communication of patient care information among healthcare providers is most efficaciously facilitated when providers all "sing from the same sheet of music." Clinical managers, department and service chiefs, and facility/system administrators must ensure that providers are using documentation formats that are universally understood by other providers in the facility/system where the relevant documentation is used. The best way to ensure this is to standardize documentation formats, requiring primary healthcare providers, for example, to use the SOAP (Subjective-Objective-Assessment-Plan) format for initial patient examination notation and the PSP (problem-status-plan) format for patient follow-up and discharge notation.

Alternatively, a facility or system may mandate the use of a common template or series of template forms for patient care documentation, on paper or in electronic formats, including hand-held tablet personal computers (PCs) and personal digital assistants (PDAs). Obviously, some degree of flexibility must be built into any standardized documentation system. However, the use of enigmatic formats or data by individual providers should be prohibited as a matter of policy. If professional colleagues cannot decipher your patient care notation, "What we have here is a failure to communicate."

Documentation Error: Failure to Use an Indelible Instrument to Record Examination, Evaluation, Diagnostic, Prognostic, or Outcome Data About a Patient Under Care

Another common documentation error involves the use of writing instruments other than indelible ink, such as pencils, erasable ink, and felt-tipped pens, by providers whose patient care entries are easily obliterated or smeared. When patient care entries are made in pencil or erasable ink, the temptation to "correct" or otherwise alter entries—especially in the face of a potential legal action—is heightened. As a preventive measure for the protection of all concerned, do not write or allow providers under your control to write patient care entries in any medium except indelible (black or dark blue) ink. Even where there is no evidence of alteration or spoliation of records in a healthcare malpractice case, an inference of negligence might be ascribed by a jury or judge to a facility in which the use of erasable notation is tolerated.

In a similar vein, always ensure that electronic patient care entries are saved on the computer before leaving the relevant software program. Administrators should systematically provide for "automatic save" features to prevent the loss or subsequent alteration of crucial patient care data when an operator leaves an electronic patient care documentation program.

Documentation Problem: Pen Runs Out of Ink Midway Through a Patient Care Entry

What do you do if, when writing a paper-based patient care entry, your pen runs out of ink? Well, obviously you must complete the entry with a second pen (hopefully with the same color ink). You should precede the second part of the entry, however, with a brief parenthetical phrase, stating that your first pen ran out of ink at that point. Be sure to initial the parenthetical comment.

The parenthetical comment is necessary to prevent a later inference of spoliation (impermissible alteration) of records in the event of any legal action involving the patient in whose record patient care activities are being documented. An example of how to document a change in writing instrument part of the way through documenting an entry appears in Exhibit 2–1.

Exhibit 2–1 Documenting a Necessary Change of Writing Instrument During a Patient Care Record Entry

Consider the case in which a registered nurse's pen runs out of ink midway through the entry of a narrative-format nursing progress note made at a shift change. The change in pens would be documented as follows:

Nov. 23, 201x/1445: Patient resting comfortably. Dyspneic breathing / (Note: Original pen ran out of ink. M.K.M., RN) / no longer observed. Normal skin color.
RR = 14/min.
(signature and title).

Documentation Problem: Line Spacing in Patient Care Record Entries

As will be elucidated in greater detail in the next chapter, spoliation or alteration of patient health records is a growing problem with serious ethical and legal implications for healthcare professionals and organizations.

One effective method that clinical managers and facility/system administrators can use to decrease the temptation on the part of providers to add information to prior entries is to establish a policy requiring that providers documenting patient care write on every line. (*Note*: In many of the illustrations throughout this book, spaces appear between lines of documentation but are interspersed solely for the purpose of highlighting different elements of the entries. Such spacing should not be construed as the recommended spacing for patient treatment documentation.)

Documentation Problem: Signing Patient Care Record Entries

By signing (or initialing) a patient care entry, a provider authenticates and acknowledges legal and professional ethical responsibility for the information contained in the entry. It goes without saying that one should have special pride in his or her signature, so providers are urged to sign patient care entries legibly and neatly. From a risk-management perspective, a legible and neat signature may also serve to create a positive impression in the minds of others reviewing the record. In the event of a subsequent healthcare malpractice proceeding involving the record, a judge and jury viewing a record with a neat signature may rightly conclude that its author was as careful and precise in caring for the patient–litigant as in signing his or her name.

Along with one's signature, the author of a patient care entry should include his or her professional title (e.g., COTA, CPO, DC, DO, LPN, MD, NP, OTR, PA, PT, PTA, RD, RN, SLP, etc.). Irrespective of how neat a signature is, a stamp with the provider's full legal name and title should be affixed in the vicinity of the signature. State or federal law, facility/system policy, and local or national customary practice may dictate inclusion of other information in a legal signature, including the provider's professional license number.

State or federal law also dictates whether a rubber stamp impression of a provider's signature or a computer-generated electronic signature constitutes a valid legal "signature." Electronic health records are discussed in greater detail in Chapter 6.

Documentation Problem: Error Correction

To err is human. To correct errors properly in patient care records is good risk management. Despite a good faith effort to document accurately the first time around, everyone will make mistakes occasionally when documenting patient care data. Mistakes can range from using an incorrect term in an entry to writing a patient's entry on a page labeled with another patient's personal data.

Individual healthcare professionals who write patient care entries, clinical managers, and facility/system administrators should develop standardized rules for correcting patient care entries in records and on other official documents. One method that is commonly used is to draw (or trace along a straightedge ruler) a single line neatly through the erroneous material and then initial it. Providers should also consider indicating the date and time of the correction, even though error correction normally is made during the same sitting as the original erroneous entry.

A basic rule that must be obeyed is to avoid hiding a mistake. Do not obliterate any patient care entry by scratching out what is written. Do not erase any entry. Similarly, the use of correction liquid to obliterate a prior entry in patient care records is a prohibited method of error correction. The purpose of patient care record error correction is to prevent a potential miscommunication of information, not to hide or obliterate what is being edited.

Even writing over an entry a second time for the innocent purpose of making lighter ink more readable is discouraged, because a patient-plaintiff 's attorney, or a judge or jury, reviewing the record at a later date may reasonably be suspicious that an improper entry alteration had occurred. Ensure that what you write in a patient's record is clear, bright, and neat the first time.

Criminologists are expert at detecting alteration of patient care record entries, and such evidence, in the face of a denial of record alteration, is devastating to a healthcare professional's credibility generally and to the defense case in healthcare malpractice proceedings. Specialists can readily distinguish the ink from two different pens, even when the color appears identical to the naked eye, and can even opine on whether entries were made at different times on the basis of penmanship and writing style.

What should a provider involved in a healthcare malpractice case say if he or she has committed an error in patient data entry correction, such as obliterating a prior entry? By all means, the provider concerned must coordinate with legal counsel on what specifically to do and say about the mistake during deposition, at trial, or in any other official proceeding. In all cases, he or she must not deny the mistake if asked about it during such proceedings. To do so would be to give false testimony—a criminal offense in most cases.

Authorities writing on the subject recommend different approaches to commenting on why error correction is being carried out. One acceptable method of correcting patient care entry errors is simply to draw through the erroneous material and initial and date the deletion, as discussed previously. Some authorities recommend the commonly-used technique of handwriting the word "error" above the correction. Others urge providers not to use the word "error" to prevent an inference of clinical negligence associated with the entry error from arising in a judge's or jury's mind. Some authorities recommends using words such as "mistake" or "mistaken entry" ("ME," if this is a recognized abbreviation), instead of "error." Still others recommend writing a brief note in the margin adjacent to the correction indicating why it was made. The most prudent approach to annotating error corrections may be to avoid add-ons altogether, so as not to create an adverse inference of sloppy patient care in the minds of judges or juries in healthcare malpractice proceedings.

Examples of acceptable techniques for patient treatment entry error correction appear in Appendix 2-B, Exhibits 2-B-1 through 2-B-2.

> The purpose of patient care notation error correction is to prevent a potential miscommunication of information, not to hide or obliterate what is being edited.

Focus on Ethics

C is a nurse practitioner in a busy private solo outpatient geriatric patient practice. When documenting patient D's history and physical examination, C inadvertently writes the data in patient E's chart. When C realizes the documentation error and the fact that no other information (except E's personal identifying information) appears on the page written on, C carefully shreds the erroneous documentation page, and replaces it with a fresh unwritten page in E's chart, then correctly documents D's information in D's chart. Has C violated any ethical or legal standards?

Documentation Error: Unauthorized and Unrecognized Abbreviations

In the busy managed care environment of contemporary patient care, nothing is more at a premium than time. Using acceptable abbreviations in patient care notation is a smart way to facilitate communication and save precious minutes that writing each and every term and phrase out longhand would entail. The selective use of abbreviations facilitates communication and improves patient care because it is easier for other providers caring for a patient being written about to scan shorter notes containing known abbreviations than to labor through longer narratives without abbreviations.

Clinicians, however, need to exercise caution when using abbreviations to ensure that others understand what information they intend to convey. To ensure uniformity and universal comprehension, clinical, facility, and system managers must develop standardized lists of approved abbreviations and require providers to use only those abbreviations. The list or lists of facility-approved abbreviations must be widely disseminated to all those personnel who do or might write, interpret, transcribe, and review patient care notation, including clinicians, students, medical records personnel, and administrative, secretarial, and clerical personnel.

Facility/system administrators should seek broad input from all potential users when formulating the lists and must ensure that approved abbreviations lists remain current. An ongoing systematic review of existing approved abbreviations is highly recommended.

Special caution must be exercised when one abbreviation may have two or more common meanings, such as "AC," for acromioclavicular, alternating current, or anterior cruciate. Similarly, abbreviations such as q.d. (every day), q.o.d. (every other day), and q.i.d. (four times a day) are so close in their makeup that they can be readily misinterpreted by other providers, and therefore should not be used in paper-based patient care documentation, as recommended by CNA in its 2006 Claims Study. If the intended meaning for such an abbreviation is not crystal clear to potential readers, then the writer must spell the word out to ensure comprehension by all.

The potential adverse consequences of using unintelligible abbreviations can be as serious as carrying out patient care in a negligent manner. If providers relying on cryptic patient care documentation misinterpret vital patient information and take injurious courses of action toward a patient as a result, then both the drafter and reader of that erroneous information may face healthcare malpractice liability.

An example of a shell rehabilitation service-approved abbreviations list appears as Appendix C.

Documentation Errors: Improper Spelling, Grammar, and the Use of Extraneous Verbiage Not Affecting Patient Care

As with illegible notation, improper word spelling and the use of incorrect grammar by healthcare professionals reflects negatively on them individually and on departments, services, facilities, and systems. These vocabulary errors may create an impression of carelessness, which, if inferred and extrapolated by judges or juries in healthcare malpractice legal cases, may contribute to findings of liability. Examples include misspelled words like "mussels" (for muscles) and "uteriss" (for uterus).

Always have readily available both a medical and standard dictionary for reference when writing patient care and related documentation. Alternatively, consider downloading a medical dictionary to your smartphone for ready use. Clinical managers and facility/system administrators should also consider developing lists of lay and medical terms that are frequently misspelled and disseminating them to staff for training use.

Regarding extraneous verbiage not affecting patient care, a basic rule of thumb to remember is that only information related to patient examination, evaluation, diagnosis, prognosis, or intervention belongs in a patient care record. As an example, it would be wholly appropriate to record in the subjective portion of a SOAP note a patient's verbalization of his or her pain symptoms. It would be inappropriate to comment in the record irrelevant information about another healthcare provider's demeanor during official exchange about patient care (e.g., "Mar. 12, 201x/0400: Called Dr. Smith regarding patient's c/o stomachache. Dr. Smith *seemed irritated about receiving the call, but* ordered Maalox for the patient p.r.n.—Regina Doe, RN") [italicized material is extraneous, and must be deleted].

Documentation Problems: Transcription Problems with Physician Orders—Examining and Intervening on Behalf of Patients Without Written Orders

Nurses and nurse practitioners, physician assistants, physical, occupational, and speech therapists, and other primary healthcare providers working in either inpatient or ambulatory care settings who read doctors' and other referring providers' preprinted or typed orders normally have no difficulty interpreting their meaning. However, handwritten orders written in haste—particularly during emergency situations—are often illegible. Healthcare professionals caring for patients pursuant to such referrals must be sure to clarify any ambiguities before carrying out orders, rather than making possibly erroneous assumptions about what is meant, to prevent patient injuries and potentially compensable events that could ripen into legal actions for healthcare malpractice.

Facility and departmental managers must establish policies that encourage providers who interpret physicians' orders to seek clarification of orders that appear ambiguous. These policies should be in writing and should be disseminated to all providers covered by their provisions. The policies should delineate appropriate methods for questioning such orders and spell out acceptable procedures for challenging suspected erroneous orders. Providers should remember to document carefully their inquiries and physician responses regarding ambiguities in diagnostic and treatment orders.

State and federal laws, facility policies, accreditation standards, and local customs govern the practice of caring for patients under verbal versus written physician's orders. Referral orders involving referring providers and consultants also raise important documentation issues. For many healthcare providers, the law requires written referral orders to treat patients referred by physicians and others for care. Even when allowed by law, clinicians such as physical therapists in the 48 of 50 direct access states who evaluate patients under verbal referral orders should always require the referring physician, dentist, or other provider to authenticate such orders expeditiously with signed written orders to enhance communication and protect both the referring provider and the clinician to whom the patient is referred. A sample form letter for requesting such orders appears in Exhibit 2–2.

Exhibit 2–2 Sample Request for Written Referral Orders to Accompany Verbal Referral Orders

Anytown Community Hospital, Anytown, USA, Physical Therapy Clinic

May 1, 201x
TO : Dr. Doe
FROM : Reginald P. Hasenfus, PT

SUBJECT : Written referral orders re Patient dx:

Dear Dr. Doe:

Please sign the enclosed referral order and return it to me in the enclosed stamped envelope so that we may complete our records and commence patient intervention for Mr. Tom Smith. Per your request during our telephonic consultation of April 29, 201x, I have examined Mr. Smith. I am enclosing the report of my examination, evaluative findings, and physical therapy diagnosis. Thank you for your prompt response.

Sincerely,
Reginald P. Hasenfus, PT, Chief Physical Therapist

Documentation Error: Untimely Documentation of Patient Care Activities

No factor contributes more to effective communication among healthcare providers simultaneously caring for patients than does the timely documentation of care. Failure to timely document important patient clinical information that other providers can use to prevent or alleviate patient suffering, or to effect speedier recovery or optimal function, is a form of professional negligence.

Ideally, timely documentation of patient care occurs concurrently with the rendition of care. This is especially facile when providers use ambulatory tablet PCs or PDAs.

In reality, however, patient care notation is often made at the end of a work shift. The further in time documentation of care occurs from the actual rendition of care or observation of a significant patient event or condition, the less accurate it becomes.

Attorneys examining healthcare providers in depositions or at trial often successfully challenge the accuracy of their documentation of patient care based on untimely notation. They persuasively argue before juries and judges that a provider's memory of critical events—like that of any percipient witness to an event—fades with the passage of time. Notation of care or patient status made hours, days, or even weeks after the fact, then, is less credible than when it is documented contemporaneously with care or observation.

Equally untimely is documentation that is made before care is actually rendered. Consider, for example, the following hypothetical situation:

> A, a clinical physical therapist at ABC General Hospital, examines patient B for a complaint of interscapular myofascial pain. As part of B's plan of care, A initiates moist heat, myofascial soft tissue mobilization, pulsed ultrasound to break up tissue adhesions, and active range of motion exercises for patient B. Before patient B is finished with her first treatment session, A completes his initial patient care note, stating in part that, "B had no adverse reaction to the initial treatment." Several minutes later, C, A's physical therapist assistant, informs A that B sustained a skin burn from the moist heat treatment. To correct his initial misimpression of patient B's tolerance of treatment, A must then either write an addendum to his original note or cross out and correct the erroneous portion of the original note. In either case, A's credibility may be diminished, and if the incident devolves into a lawsuit, a jury or judge might be less likely generally to believe A's testimony about patient B's care than if the erroneous comment about patient B's status had not been improperly and incorrectly written in advance.

The physical therapist in this example could have prevented the loss of credibility regarding his testimony about patient B's overall care by having waited until patient B completed her initial treatment session to document B's postintervention status.

Occasionally, providers will be required to document entries that are made some time after care has been rendered or after important information about a patient's status has already been observed. Such a late entry may necessarily occur when the provider may not have ready access to the patient's record or, as in the previous hypothetical situation, when additional clinically pertinent information about the patient becomes available only after the initial note is completed. A late entry should always be labeled as an "addendum" or "follow-on entry" to avoid a later inference that spoliation (improper alteration of the patient's record) occurred. Also, a late entry should be labeled with the date and time that it is written. If a late entry does not build on the entry immediately preceding it, then some reference to the prior entry being amended must be made in the body of the late entry.

An example of how to document correctly the original and late entries illustrated in the previous hypothetical situation appears in Exhibit 2–3.

Exhibit 2–3 Example of Documenting a Necessary Late Patient Care Entry at ABC General Hospital Physical Therapy Department

Oct. 31, 201x

S: 49 y o F, dx: right interscapular myofascial pain syndrome, referred by Dr. Johansen of Pain Clinic for "evaluation and appropriate treatment." Hx of R FOOSH Oct. 20, 201x. No fx in RUE, acc to x-ray report in pt.'s OPR, dtd. Oct. 21, 201x. Pt. rates her localized pain (see diagram) as 6/10, and constant. No rad, neg. sensory sx, acc to pt. Meds: Motrin, Robaxin. Neg. prior hx. Pt. is homemaker and avocational painter.

O: GMT NL, BUE. FAROM BUE and C sp. Reflexes 2+/symm., BUE. SLT intact BUE and C & T sp. Neg. deformity; 12 trigger points of pain along sup. and med. R scapular border. Posture NL.

A: Myofascial pain syndrome, R interscapular region, secondary to R upper quarter trauma 10 days ago. ADL dysfunction (homemaking and painting activities).

P: MH, US, myofascial mobilization, AROM B Scapula and C & T sp., in clinic X 5. Pt. verbalizes decreased local sx. From 6/10 to 4/10 p/ initial rx. No adverse reaction to rx.

G: Decrease pain sx to 0–1/10 X 2–3 wks, so that pt. can carry out independent pain-free ADL; prevent recurrence through pt. education.

ADDENDUM: Oct. 31, 201x/1400: Initial entry of this date incorrectly stated that pt. had no adverse reaction to initial care. Approx. 5 min. subsequent to note being written at 1330, pt. reportedly sustained a skin burn from MH over R medial scapular border, as reported to me by Carl Modality, PTA. Burn appears bright red, painful, small 2" diam. unbroken blister. I called Dr. Johansen and reported findings; pt. treated w/ ice pack X 20 min, per Dr. Johansen VO. Pain and redness completely resolved. F/U w/ Dr. Johansen in AM or p.r.n. earlier.

—Bob Therapist, PT

Documentation Error: Identifying or Filing an Incident Report in the Patient Care Record

Patient, visitor, staff, vendor, and other-party injuries unfortunately will occur from time to time in healthcare settings, regardless of precautions taken by clinical managers, clinicians, and support staff. When such nosocomial injuries occur, careful objective documentation of information that the provider writing about the injury perceives is critically important. Careful, complete documentation of an injury serves at least three purposes: (1) to promote optimal quality care to the injured party, (2) to serve the risk management function of protecting the facility from unwarranted liability exposure, and (3) to form the basis for further training of staff members to try to prevent similar incidents in the future.

Whenever any adverse event involving actual or potential injury to a patient, visitor, staff member, or other person occurs, a formal incident report should be completed and forwarded through the clinical manager to a centralized risk-management office for review and retention. An incident report also must be completed whenever a medication error occurs or when a patient or visitor makes a formal complaint about a facility, system, or its staff.

Administrators and clinical managers should educate their staffs that the completion of an incident report under such circumstances is the norm and will not, in and of itself, constitute a stigma against any provider potentially responsible for an adverse event. Staff members should also be educated as to why an incident report is so critically important. Because memories fade relatively quickly after an event is perceived, it is vital to document right away what happened to an injured party.

Writers of these reports, clinical managers, and facility/system administrators can feel secure in knowing that incident reports, like other quality improvement or attorney-work product documents, normally enjoy qualified immunity from release to patients, their attorneys, and others seeking to obtain them. However, because incident reports necessarily contain more detailed administrative information than a concomitant patient care note concerning care rendered to an injured party, they should not be filed in the injured party's patient care record.

Also, to avoid drawing a patient's or attorney's attention to the fact that an incident report has been filed, providers must be careful not to mention in the patient care record that an incident report has been filed. This precaution is not advocating "hiding the ball." Documentation of the existence of an incident report has no place in a patient care record because an incident report contains purely administrative and not clinical information.

Advice on techniques for designing and drafting incident reports and suggestions about their contents appear in Chapter 6.

Documentation Problem: Failing to Delineate Patient Care Rendered or Identify Clinical Information Supplied by Another Provider

Not every observation or finding described by a clinician in a patient examination, evaluation, or intervention note concerns observations or findings that the clinician perceived firsthand. Very often, other health-care professionals, support staff, and other persons supply clinically pertinent information about a patient that is incorporated into primary documentation of care. Patient care carried out by another provider as well as clinical information supplied by another person to the writer of a patient care note should be clearly attributed to the source person.

Failure to denote another person's responsibility for clinical information supplied to the writer of a patient care note may result in legal responsibility being ascribed exclusively to the note writer for the information at issue. This may be the case even when the information clearly could not have emanated from the writer, for example, where a surgeon or radiologist furnishes information about a patient's medical status to a nurse, physical or occupational therapist, or other nonphysician provider caring for the patient.

Consider the following hypothetical case:

X, a staff occupational therapist at Anytown General Hospital, conducts an initial musculoskeletal evaluation of patient P, pursuant to a proper written order from Dr. Z. Patient P's diagnosis is right carpal tunnel syndrome, status post-carpal tunnel release seven days ago. Patient P is referred for "evaluation and appropriate exercises." During her evaluation of patient P, X telephones Dr. Z for consultation, after patient P reveals to X that she fell onto her outstretched right hand two days postoperatively and is now experiencing local sharp pain at the proximal thenar eminence. X suspects a carpal fracture. Patient P's chart contains no information about recent right wrist radiographs. Dr. Z advises X that she just examined patient P yesterday and ordered x-rays of her right wrist, which were negative. Dr. Z tells X to proceed with postoperative range of motion exercises. X documents in her evaluation note that patient P's right wrist x-rays were normal, without ascribing responsibility for the information to Dr. Z. X also fails to document Dr. Z's verbal instructions to her to proceed with treatment. X proceeds with treatment, which consists of home active exercises. On her one-week recheck, patient P's right proximal wrist pain has increased significantly and she is tender to palpation over the scaphoid bone. X walks to the radiology department, where she reviews patient P's prior right wrist x-rays with Dr. R, a radiology resident. Dr. R had just officially read patient P's x-rays and documented the results two days ago; they show a scaphoid fracture. When X reveals this finding to patient P, patient P becomes infuriated with X over the erroneous prior reading of her radiograph and threatens to sue. Even though Dr. Z most probably will concede that he misread patient P's radiographs and communicated to X that they were normal, an ambiguity still exists in X's initial evaluation note, in which it appears that X personally read patient P's radiographs as normal. This misinterpretation of X's evaluation note could have easily been prevented had X documented patient P's radiographic findings in the objective section of her note as follows: "X-rays of R wrist taken Mar. 19, 201x, by Dr. Z and read as normal. (Information obtained telephonically from Dr. Z on Mar. 20, 201x.)" The following phrase should also have appeared in the assessment portion of X's initial note: "P. cleared by Dr. Z for AROM exercises."

Similar misinterpretations over who is responsible for patient care or diagnostic information also can occur when assistants, aides, residents, interns, and students on clinical affiliations relate clinical information to providers who are privileged to document in patient care records, and the writer fails to denote who actually provided the care or furnished the information.

For example, consider the following hypothetical situation:

A physical therapist assistant administering therapeutic exercises to a rehabilitation patient relates to the supervising physical therapist that the patient displayed anterior shoulder pain during active arm exercises. The proper course of action for the supervising physical therapist (who is not present at the scene) is to annotate that finding in a progress note and credit the physical therapist assistant as the source of the information. Such a note might appear as follows:

Dec. 23, 201x/1900 P: 67 y o M, dx: s/p R CVA w/ residual L UE weakness.

S: Shawn Jones, PTA, reported telephonically that pt. c/o increased L ant. shoulder pain with PNF; no apparent subluxation, swelling, or other objective signs reported. I was at another location. Directed Mr. Jones to d/c exercises for now and instruct pt. and wife to cont. w/ MH or CP, according to pt. preference, p.r.n.

P: Will reexamine pt. this PM for new L UE pain complaint.

—Philomena Therapist, PT

Whenever a primary healthcare provider receives and documents clinical information about an adverse change in a patient's condition derived from another professional or support person, the primary provider becomes obligated to reexamine the patient expeditiously or risk professional negligence-based healthcare malpractice liability exposure for patient injuries for the negligent failure to appropriately monitor the patient.

Documentation Error: Blaming or Disparaging Another Provider in the Patient Care Record

Information that disparages another healthcare provider, or blames any provider for a patient's condition—either expressly or by implication—has no place in the patient care record. Such information has no clinical relevance to patient care. One type of entry often seen in patient care records that has an implication of blame is notation that documents missed patient appointments.

Consider the following hypothetical situation:

Patient Y underwent an arthroscopic debridement and repair of her torn left medial meniscus yesterday. At ABC Hospital, postoperative arthroscopic knee procedure patients go to physical therapy one day preoperatively for preoperative examination and patient education about the postoperative exercise program. In this case, a miscommunication between the orthopedic ward and physical therapy prevented patient Y from being seen preoperatively. Although all three providers involved—the orthopedic surgeon, the charge nurse for the orthopedic ward, and the orthopedic physical therapist—could give in to the temptation to document patient Y's missed preoperative physical therapy appointment defensively, it would be unproductive and perhaps inaccurate to cast aspersions on each other for the mistake. Inappropriate entries in this case would include the following three examples:

Example 1: Apr. 1, 201x/1400

P: One-day post-op L arthroscopic medial meniscus debridement and repair.

S: Minimal swelling; no drainage. Pt. reluctant to do isometric quadriceps sets. *PT neglected to see pt. for pre-op teaching.*

P: To PT today for post-op rehab per protocol.

G: D/C crutches in 1 wk; FFAROM L knee X 2–4 wks; I pain-free ADL X 6–8 wks.

—Otto Ortho, MD

Example 2: Apr. 1, 201x/1500

  S: 32 y o M, computer programmer, s/p L arthroscopic medial meniscus debridement and repair yesterday. To clinic via w/c. Referred for post-op rehab per protocol. Meds: Tylenol p.r.n. (none since 11 AM today).

  O: Alert; seems disturbed over his missed app't for pre-op education. In bulky dressing, removed, no drainage. AAROM, L knee: 0/65 degrees, min. swelling. Neurovascular system intact. Rest of lower quarter screen WNL.

  A: s/p L arthroscopic medial meniscus debridement and repair yesterday. Ready for post-op rehab; crutch walking PWB (50%). Note: *Missed preop app't was result of the ward failing to send down a pre-op consult.*

  P: CW today, begin QS, SLR, AAROM; progress per protocol. Pt. is I on crutches, at approximately 50% PWB, level and stairs; understood and safely carried out all instructed activities.

STG: D/C crutches in 1 wk; FFAROM L knee X 2–4 wks.

LTG: I pain-free ADL X 6–8 wks.

—**Ron Therapist, PT**

Example 3: Apr. 1, 201x/1415

  P: One-day post-op L arthroscopic medial meniscus debridement and repair.

  S: Dr. Ortho just ordered pt. to PT today for post-op rehab. Pt. visibly upset p/ Dr. visit because of missed pre-op PT eval. app't. *It was my fault that pt. didn't get to PT pre-op. I saw Dr. Ortho's standing pre-op order but forgot to send pt. to PT because I was involved w/ six other admissions. Sorry!*

  P: To PT now in w/c for post-op rehab and crutch gait trg. PWB (50%) per protocol.

  G: I CW PWB X 1 day, I pain management, prevent wound infection, return to work sx-free.

—**Regina Smith, RN**

The three hypothetical patient care notes given previously illustrate several important points. Dr. Ortho should not have displayed his anger over the missed preoperative teaching appointment in front of the patient. He also should not have documented in his progress note that the physical therapist was negligent in failing to see the patient preoperatively. (This conjecture was, in fact, inaccurate.)

Dr. Ortho's reaction to the patient's missed appointment and the documentation of his speculation as to its cause started a chain reaction of patient dissatisfaction and defensive documentation by other providers on the team that was irrelevant, disruptive to patient care, and unproductive. The end result may well be (depending on the outcomes of this patient's care) that the patient files a complaint, claim, or even a legal and/ or administrative action because of what occurred. If that would occur, then the defensive documentation illustrated earlier would be very helpful in support of the patient's healthcare malpractice case.

Just as Dr. Ortho and Mr. Therapist should not have blamed physical therapy and nursing, respectively, for the missed appointment in the patient's care record, Ms. Smith should not have conceded blame for the incident in the patient's record. Again, her admission has no clinical relevance and, therefore, no place in the patient care record.

Problems of this type are best addressed informally between members of the patient care team in the setting of an interdisciplinary quality management committee meeting. The focus of such a meeting is primarily on how to resolve the problem, not on targeting individuals. If more formal action is required, then the surgeon or another team member should initiate an incident report, wherein reasons for the missed appointment can be more freely detailed. Of course, an incident report would be required if the patient suffered injury as a result of the missed appointment. The incident report, as a quality assurance/improvement or attorney work product document, is normally immune from release to the patient or the patient's attorney under state or federal law.

Even in an incident report, however, a provider is not free to defame another provider by making a false accusation that damages the defamed provider's professional reputation in the eyes of others in the relevant healthcare community. Purely personal defamatory remarks are legally actionable as intentional torts (wrongs).

Defamation has two varieties: libel and slander. Written defamatory remarks about another provider, such as might appear in a patient care record, incident report, or other document, constitute "libel." Also included within the definition of libel are defamatory statements made on computer, videotape, or other relatively permanent media. Spoken defamation is called "slander." If a defendant is found liable for defamation, then the damages might include not only compensatory money damages for loss of the victim's personal and professional reputation, but also punitive, or exemplary, damages intended to punish a wrongdoer. In many states, the defendant may be personally responsible for payment of the judgment in such a case, where the defendant's insurer is statutorily relieved of responsibility for indemnification for judgments involving malicious intentional torts and/or punitive damages.

Defamation: A communication to a third party of an untrue statement about a person that damages or defames the person's good reputation in the community. Although normally a person claiming to be defamed must prove any losses suffered as a result of the defamation, damages may be presumed, and may not need to be proven, for victims who are professionals and business persons. The two classifications of defamation are as follows:

- Slander: Oral defamation
- Libel: Written, pictorial, and other more permanent modes of defamation

Documentation Error: Expressing Personal Feelings About a Patient or Patient Family Member or Significant Other in the Patient Care Record

Just as patient care documentation entries can disparage healthcare providers, inappropriate statements written about patients in their records may also constitute actionable defamation. Healthcare providers documenting patient examinations, evaluations, or interventions must exercise special caution to avoid making inappropriate personal comments about patients under their care. For example, actual observed attributions such as "malingerer," "supratentorial symptoms," "manipulator," and "pseudo-intellectual" are all inappropriate. Such comments, if discovered by the patient, will justifiably sour the patient–professional relationship and make the patient more litigation prone to healthcare malpractice and defamation causes of action. In such a case, the healthcare provider will be in the nearly impossible position of trying to establish at trial during the defense case that the documentation in issue accurately characterized the patient.

Despite the fear of a defamation action, a healthcare provider is ethically obligated to document findings that negate a patient's assertions of symptoms. This, however, must be done very carefully. Statements such as "objective examination normal" and "palpation, even to light skin touch, results in severe pain response by patient" are, if accurate, more appropriate for documentation in patient care records. More risky, but perhaps still appropriate, comments are ones such as evaluative conclusions that state, "Rule out subjective exaggeration of symptoms, based on normal objective findings," and "Rule out secondary gain." Conclusions based on conjecture, such as "Objective findings do not justify subjective complaints," are inappropriate and dangerous and must be avoided.

Providers must also be vigilant when they transcribe statements made by patients during examinations and interventions. Any statement made by a patient that is documented in the patient care record must appear in quotation marks. For example, if a patient says to a physical therapist during an examination for a complaint of work-related low back pain that his back does not hurt him now, then the therapist should quote the patient, rather than paraphrase the patient's remark, in the subjective section of the evaluation note. When documenting such a statement that is clearly contrary to the patient's self-interest, the provider should have the patient confirm the statement before writing it in the patient care record. Although it may seem to be defensive healthcare, consider having a witness present when the patient confirms such a statement. Ethically, however, such a statement requires documentation in the patient care record, because it is clinically pertinent information about the patient.

In the rare case in which a patient plainly asserts that he or she is falsifying symptoms (i.e., committing fraud) to bolster a legal case or to dupe an insurance company or workers' compensation board, the provider should immediately report that finding to his or her supervisor, organizational administrator, or legal counsel for further action.

Documentation Suggestion: Document Observations and Findings Objectively

Subjective information belongs exclusively in the subjective ("S") section of a patient care note. Clinical information documented in other sections of the note ("O," "A," and "P") must be written in objective, unambiguous, and, to the extent possible, quantifiable terms to promote clear, effective communication with other providers. Providers should avoid documenting ambiguous conclusions about a patient's status, such as "appears within normal limits," "apparent muscle tightness," and "tolerated treatment well," as well as ambiguous intervention plans, such as "routine strengthening exercises," and "conservative measures."

Documentation Suggestion: Document with Specificity

Similar to clinical information that is ambiguous and lacks objectivity is information that lacks specificity. When generalizations are made or when information that clearly can and should be quantified is not, providers miss an important opportunity to communicate effectively about their patients to other providers.

For example, if an occupational therapist conducting two-point discrimination sensory testing of a patient's hand writes "within normal limits," then other providers reading the findings can only guess at their meaning. The preferred way of documenting such findings would be to quantify in standard terms (here, millimeters) the patient's discrimination of two static or moving sharp points and report results (pictorially and numerically) for specific locations on specific fingers.

Another example concerns a hypothetical physician's assistant conducting reflex testing of a patient during a neurologic examination. If the physician assistant reports "reflexes WNL," then other providers reading the note have no clue as to which reflexes were tested or what "WNL" means. More specific and meaningful would be the following report: "Biceps, triceps, and brachioradialis reflexes 2+/symmetrical/brisk in both upper limbs."

Documentation Error: Recording Hearsay (Secondhand Information) as Fact

Documenting hearsay as if it were fact is a common and dangerous practice that can leave healthcare providers in a position of increased vulnerability to healthcare malpractice and defamation liability exposure. Hearsay is a legal term of art used to describe any extrajudicial (out-of-court) statement offered as evidence in court for the truth of the matter asserted in it. Regarding patient care documentation, hearsay describes a statement made by one person and adopted as fact by another person. That is, hearsay describes secondhand input.

Take, for example, the case in which a physical therapist, P, who intervenes for patients bedside on hospital wards, enters patient Q's room. Q is a 65-year-old male patient, status post-left cerebrovascular accident, with right hemiparesis and poor standing balance. Q is not yet ambulatory. On entering Q's room, P notices Q lying on the floor next to his bed, moaning. The bed rail is down. Sitting on a chair next to the bed is Q's wife, R. When P asks R what happened, she replies, "The bed rail was down and he rolled out of bed." P calls loudly for help; Q is examined by Dr. S and found to be unhurt, except for two minor bruises on his right elbow and right femoral greater trochanter. Q's status would be correctly described in progress notes by P and Dr. S as follows:

June 25, 201x/1425

P: L CVA; R hemiparesis; bedside PT pt.

S: Found lying on floor next to bed. Dr. S examined pt. and stated pt. is "Fine, except for two small bruises, one on R elbow, one on R greater trochanter." Dr. S ordered PT held for today.

P: Hold PT today, recheck status in AM.

G: Progress to standing X 1 wk

—**Endie Tee, PT**

June 25, 201x/1428

P: L CVA; R hemiparesis.

S: Mr. Tee, PT, reported that pt. found on floor next to bed. Examination WNL, except for two small bruises, one on R elbow, one on R greater trochanter.

P: Hold PT for today; monitor V/S q 4 hrs X 24 hrs. Re-examine in AM

—**Vigil Lant, MD**

Note that each provider only documented as firsthand the clinical information that he personally perceived. The physical therapist and physician each correctly attributed hearsay information provided by the other appropriately in his note. Also note that neither provider made mention in patient care documentation of how patient Q might have alighted from his bed. That information was correctly excluded from their documentation. Such information should instead be documented in an incident report. Because Q's wife supplied that information, her hearsay statements must be appropriately recorded in the incident report. This example will be revisited in Chapter 6, when incident report documentation is discussed in greater detail.

Another example of hearsay involves information related by a patient presenting for examination with incomplete prior documentation of the patient's status. Consider, for instance, the case in which a physical therapist is examining a patient pursuant to a written physician referral, with a diagnosis of left lateral (humeral) epicondylitis. The therapist does not have any reports about radiographs. The patient volunteers that the referring physician took radiographs of the left elbow and read them as normal. If the therapist relies on that information in his or her examination, evaluation, and diagnosis, it must be properly attributed to the patient as the source of the information. It would, therefore, be incorrect for the therapist to write "x-ray WNL" as part of the examination. Instead, the therapist would correctly document in his or her patient care notation as follows, including reference to patient as source for information about the left elbow x-ray and the patient's allergic status:

Aug. 5, 201x

S: 45 y o F, dx: L lat. epicondylitis; referred for "evaluation and appropriate Rx."

O: Alert, cooperative. FAROM BUE; GMT NL BUE. Neg. swelling peri-L lat. epicondyle. SLT intact BUE. Min. TTP L proximal lat. epicondyle. Mod. c/o pain L lat. epicondyle w/ resisted L wrist extension and passive L wrist flexion. Per pt., x-ray of L elbow, taken by Dr. X, Aug. 3, 201x, reported to her as WNL by Dr. X. (No report available; Dr. X and staff on vacation.)

A: L lat. epicondylitis.

P: HCP X 5 (pt. reports "no allergy to HC"), gentle AROM, progress to PREs. No objective signs, or patient complaint of problems, with Rx.

G: Decrease sx 25% X 2 wks, I pain-free ADL (cooking, tennis) X 2–4 wks, prevent recurrence through ADL hints.

—John P. Doe, PT

Documentation Suggestion: Exercise Special Caution When Countersigning Another Provider's, Student's, or Intern's Patient Care Notation

Staff physicians, clinical preceptors, and other primary healthcare providers are frequently called on to serve as clinical instructors and preceptors for health professions students. In that role, providers routinely countersign patient care notation made by students under their supervision. In most cases, such authentication is required to make the student's documentation legally acceptable. Providers who countersign another persons' patient care notes are urged to proofread carefully what is written because, like a guarantor who cosigns for a loan for another person, the countersigning healthcare professional assumes legal responsibility for the information contained in the note.

If the supervising clinical instructor or mentor observes incomplete or inaccurate information in a student's or intern's patient care note, then the supervisor is obligated to correct the note before signing it. This may be done by having the student correct discrepancies in the documentation or, as supervisor, by correcting the note and initialing the modifications made. Once countersigned, a student or intern's patient care note is legally adopted by the supervising healthcare professional as his or her own note. The preceptor then shares legal responsibility for what is written therein.

> Once countersigned, a student or intern's patient care note is legally adopted by the supervising healthcare professional as his or her own note. The preceptor then shares legal responsibility for what is written therein.

Documentation Error: Failure to Document a Patient's Informed Consent to Examination and Intervention

The concept of informed consent recognizes the fundamental ethical and human rights principle that every adult patient with full mental capacity has the right of control over healthcare decision-making and must be given sufficient clinical disclosure information by a healthcare provider to make an informed choice. For many procedures, such as surgical procedures and administration of anesthesia, state statutory law spells out documentation requirements that serve as ethically and legally sufficient evidence of a patient's informed consent to intervention. For most routine healthcare interventions, however, there are no statutory formats to comply with to document patients' informed consent. Providers, therefore, should consider devising their own formats for documenting patients' informed consent to routine healthcare interventions. Informed consent to treatment generally, and suggested formats for documenting informed consent in particular, are discussed in greater detail in Chapter 4.

Documentation Suggestion: Document Thoroughly Patient/ Family/Significant Other Understanding of, and Safe Compliance with, Discharge, Home Care, and Follow-up Instructions

In a managed care environment, characterized by diminished reimbursement for healthcare services, the legal standards of care for physicians, nurses, physical, occupational, and speech therapists, orthotists and prosthetists, and other healthcare providers includes the issuance of written homecare instructions to patients on discharge from the hospital or from outpatient care. Providers are urged to retain master copies of standardized homecare instructions given routinely to patients and/or families/ significant others caring for patients at home. These forms should be an integral part of a clinic procedures manual.

Service chiefs and risk managers should ensure that staff clinicians provide written, personalized homecare instructions to every patient. If issuance of these written homecare instructions becomes a standard clinical practice, then even in the absence of documentation of their issuance, providers testifying at a healthcare malpractice trial years after their issuance can truthfully testify that the issuance of written homecare instructions is universal and customary practice. Such evidence of customary practice, even when the provider cannot recall a specific case or patient, is usually admissible as substantive evidence of compliance with the custom in an individual case.

As with informed consent, a provider should document that a patient and/or family member or significant other understands, safely carries out, and accepts responsibility for compliance with a home program of care. The provider should also document any special precautions or limitations on the patient's activities as well as follow-up care instructions. It may constitute patient abandonment to not offer necessary follow-up to a homecare patient.

Such documentation in a patient discharge note might appear as follows:

Oct. 31, 201x

P: L CVA, R UE hemiparesis.

S: Alert, cooperative, independent in all relevant ADL, FAROM w/ NL gross muscle test BUE. SLT intact BUE. Reflexes 2+/symm. BUE. Normal R UE proprioception.

P: Discharge to home. Written instructions for home exercises, including PNF and AROM exercises, issued to pt. Pt. to stop program if severe pain, swelling, or loss of sensation occurs, and report symptoms to me immediately. Pt. understands all, agrees to comply with program as outlined in handout, and safely demonstrated all recommended home exercises. Follow-up 2–3 wks or p.r.n earlier, as needed.

G: Increase R UE strength to enable pt. to perform pre stroke household duties within 1–2 mos.

—J. Ray, OTR/L

Documentation of homecare follow-up instructions issued to a patient/family member/significant other responsible for home care on discharge.

List of required elements:

- Written homecare instructions issued
- Patient/family member/significant other advised about any special precautions or limitations associated with the homecare program
- Instructions for follow-up reexamination, as indicated
- Written documentation that patient/family member/significant other understands and consents to the homecare program, acknowledges responsibility for compliance with it, and demonstrates the ability to carry it out competently and safely.

It may constitute patient abandonment to not offer necessary follow-up to a homecare patient.

Documentation Suggestion: Carefully Document a Patient's Noncompliance with Provider Directives or Orders

Documenting patients' noncompliance with care is an important risk-management tool to protect healthcare providers individually and their employing healthcare organizations from healthcare malpractice liability in the event that a claim or lawsuit ensues, resulting from alleged injuries incident to care. Providers should carefully document noncompliance events involving patients under their care, such as refusal to comply with the facility's "no smoking" policy or to comply with dietary restrictions, refusal to ask for ambulatory assistance where the patient cannot ambulate independently (with or without assistive devices), refusal to use ambulatory assistive devices when ordered, refusal to take medications as ordered, or to carry out exercises or other important interventions. Careful, thorough, objective, nondefensive documentation including specific therapeutic orders violated and dates, times, and circumstances of patient noncompliance should be included in such notation.

Documentation Suggestion: Carefully Document a Patient's or Family Member's/Significant Other's Possible Contributory Negligence Related to Alleged Patient Injuries or Lack of Progress

In some instances, health professional negligence can be inferred or presumed if patients are injured under circumstances in which they normally would not suffer injury, absent a provider's probable negligence. Such circumstances might include patient falls while transferring or ambulating, falling from the bed onto the floor, medication overdoses, burns while under heat or ice treatment, and tissue ischemia from tight compression garments, casts, or orthoses.

Under the legal concept of *res ipsa loquitur*, professional negligence might be presumed against a healthcare provider in the previous situations unless there is documented evidence that the patient or a family member/significant other caused or contributed to the patient's injuries. Like everyone, a patient can be contributorily negligent (i.e., fail to conform to the standards required by law for his or her own safety and protection from harm).

Healthcare providers must carefully document a patient's refusal to comply with recommendations and instructions, as well as a patient's misuse or tampering with exercise equipment or other therapeutic devices, such as electric heating pads or neuromuscular stimulation devices. When a patient is contributorily negligent and suffers injury as a result, the patient cannot normally invoke *res ipsa loquitur* as an aid to proving a case of healthcare malpractice.

CHAPTER SUMMARY

Documentation of patient care is as important as the rendition of care itself. This chapter introduces patient care documentation management and methodology. The most important reason to document patient examination, evaluation, diagnosis, prognosis, intervention, and follow-up care is to record pertinent clinical information about the patient and communicate it to other healthcare providers caring for the patient, now or in the future. Secondary reasons justifying effective patient care documentation include, among others, identifying staff training needs, justifying reimbursement for care, and serving the risk-management function of memorializing the examination and interventions performed on a patient's behalf and by whom. A suggested standardized format for patient examinations/evaluations is the SOAPG (subjective-objective-assessment-plan-functional goals) format. For progress and discharge notes, healthcare providers and organizations are urged to consider using the more streamlined PSP (problem-status-plan) problem-oriented format for recording patient care information. This chapter includes detailed discussion of 25 selected documentation problems, errors, and suggestions for improving patient care documentation. The goal that providers must strive for is to document findings and observations of clinical relevance accurately, clearly, comprehensively, and in a timely manner. Documentation should be objective, specific, and nondefensive. The end result of a carefully designed documentation program—whether handwritten, in electronic format, or a combination of both—is optimal quality patient care.

> The end result of a carefully designed documentation program is optimal quality patient care.

REFERENCES AND SUGGESTED READINGS

Blount E. M.D.s Who Mind Their P's and Q's Shouldn't Misplace Their Modifiers. *Wall Street Journal.* 1999; Jan 27:B1.

Brooks ML. *Exploring Medical Language*, 7th ed. St. Louis, MO: Mosby-Elsevier, Inc; 2009.

Centers for Medicare & Medicaid Services (CMS), U.S. Department of Health and Human Services. Homepage. Accessed June 15, 2011 from http//www.cms.gov

Clifton DW. Tolerated treatment well may no longer be tolerated. *PT: Magazine of Physical Therapy.* 1995; 3(10):24–27.

CNA Physical Therapy Claims Study, 2006.

Direct Access State Laws Table. Alexandria, VA: American Physical Therapy Association; 2010.

Guidelines for Physical Therapy Documentation. Alexandria, VA: American Physical Therapy Association; 2004.

Jette DU. On tolerating treatment well. *PT: Magazine of Physical Therapy.* 1996; 4(4):13.

Kettenbach G. *Writing SOAP Notes*, 3rd ed. Philadelphia: FA Davis Co; 2004.

Kollenberg LO. Payment depends on documentation. *Biomechanics.* 1998; February: 39–43.

Pagano MP. *Authoring Patient Records.* Sudbury, MA: Jones and Bartlett, Inc; 2011.

Pierson FM, Fairchild S. *Principles and Techniques of Patient Care*, 2nd ed. Philadelphia: WB Saunders Co; 2010.

Scott RW. Incident reports: Protecting the record. *PT: Magazine of Physical Therapy.* 1996; 4(9):24–25.

United States Census Bureau. *The 2011 Statistical Abstract. The National Data Book.* Modified January 20, 2011. Health and Nutrition: Health Expenditures. Accessed June 15, 2011 from http:www.census.gov/compendia/statab/cats/health_nutrition/health_expenditures.html

REVIEW CASE STUDIES

1. You are the Director of Medical Records for ABC Hospital. A staff rehabilitation professional asks your opinion on giving greater emphasis to critically important details in the narrative sections of incident reports filed within the system by placing such important details in quotation marks. How do you respond?

2. Dr. A, a neurosurgeon at XYZ Medical Center, refuses to adhere to the facility's required patient care documentation format, which consists of the SOAPG (subjective-objective-assessment-plan-goals) format for new patient evaluations and the PSP

(problem-status-plan) format for treatment, progress, and reevaluation notation. As service chief or hospital administrator, how would you convince Dr. A to conform to this practice standard?

DISCUSSION: REVIEW CASE STUDIES

1. The staff rehabilitation professional is correct in opining that witness statements must appear in quotation marks in the narrative sections of incident reports. To merely paraphrase witnesses' statements would do a disservice to all persons and entities affected by an adverse incident, including patients, providers, quality and safety management committees, administrators, attorneys, and others. However, other information should probably not be placed in quotation marks. Authorities state that the overuse of quotation marks in writing may be indicative of stress on the part of the writer. (Reference: Carton B. Why does "everybody" now put "everything" in quotation marks? *Wall Street Journal.* March 15, 1999: A1.) In the case of an adverse patient incident in a healthcare facility that may ripen into a claim or lawsuit, an inference of stressed-out healthcare professionals made by a patient-plaintiff 's attorney at trial may be extended by a sympathetic jury into a presumption of substandard healthcare delivery. Avoid the overuse of quotation marks in patient care documentation.

2. There are several incremental approaches that can be used to obtain Dr. A's compliance with institutional standards. The best initial approach would probably be to schedule a formal meeting with Dr. A and the service chief and the hospital administrator to educate Dr. A about the need for standardized patient care documentation that is readily comprehensible by other healthcare professionals in the facility. Such a system, and only such a system, fulfills the primary purpose of patient care documentation: to communicate pertinent clinical information about patients expeditiously to other healthcare providers having a need to know.

If noncompliance persists, formal counseling should be undertaken, with appropriate documentation in Dr. A's provider-activity file. As a last and drastic resort, retention of clinical privileges can be conditioned on Dr. A's compliance with this vital practice standard. Before adverse action affecting privileges occurs, however, Dr. A should be advised by the hospital attorney about the administrative consequences of an adverse action affecting clinical privileges (i.e., reporting of the action to the National Practitioner Data Bank).

For the Suggested Answer Framework to the Focus on Ethics, please refer to Appendix D.

2-A

Additional Examples of Patient Care Documentation Formats

Exhibit 2-A-1 Sample SOAP Patient Initial Visit Note

The following is a physical therapist's initial note for an outpatient seen in a private practice setting:

ABC Physical Therapy Clinic, Anytown, USA

May 1, 201x

S: 47 y o M, college math professor, dx: chronic LBP syndrome, referral for "evaluation and treatment." Pt. states that his pain is in the midline lumbar spine, is constant, occasionally radiates across R buttock to R post thigh just above the knee, worse w/ sitting and prolonged standing, better w/ rest, esp. sleeping on L side. No c/o sensory systems. Neg. B/B. Hx of sx for 1 yr, since fall on ice onto back w he shoveling snow at home (Apr. 19, 201x). Spent 10 days in hospital, undergoing lumbar traction and WFE, with initial success. Intermittent OP rx since then. (Records w/ pt., reviewed.) No prior back hx, no subsequent injury. Med. hx: adult-onset DM, controlled by diet, stomach ulcer, GB surgery, Feb. 1998. Meds: Ibuprofen 800 mg t.i.d prn, Tagamet.

O: Alert, cooperative. Does not appear to be in acute distress. X-ray, L spine, Apr. 23, 201x: mild facet DJD, otherwise WNL. GMT NL

SLE, AROM BLE. L spine AROM: FB full, BB 1/2 w/ pain in midline L spine, SB full B. Reflexes 2+/symm. BLE. SLT intact, symm. BLE and L spine. Neg. SLR to 85 degrees B; neg. Fabere B. SIJ screen WNL. Neg. spasm, TTP, deformity, L spine. Posture WNL. Gait WNL.

A: Chronic LBP syndrome, mild L spine DJD, probable lumbar extension dysfunction, r/o HNP.

P: MH today in clinic, F/B prone active extension exercises, 10–15 reps, postural, lifting, and sleeping hints. I/C obtained for Rx. No observed adverse reaction to Rx. Cont. w/ home program of MH p.r.n. a/ or p/ extension exercises as above, tid. X 30 days. Understands all; no questions. Schedule for back school. F/U p/ re-eval. w/ Dr. Brown, or four wks, or p.r.n. earlier.

—**Ron Therapist, PT**

Exhibit 2-A-2 Sample Hx-SOAP Patient Evaluation Note

The following is a physical therapist's initial note for a hospitalized inpatient evaluated in a small community hospital:

Anytown Community Hospital, Anytown, USA
Physical Therapy Clinic
May 1, 201x

Hx: Dx: Chronic LBP syndrome (Dr. Brown). Hx of sx for 1 yr, since fall on ice onto back while shoveling snow at home (Apr. 19, 201x). Spent 10 days in hospital, undergoing lumbar traction, WFE, MH, and US, with initial success. Intermittent OP Rx since then. (Records w/ pt. and reviewed.) No prior back hx, no subsequent injury. Med. hx: AODM, controlled by diet, stomach ulcer, GB surgery, Feb. 1998.

S: 47 y o M, college math professor, referred for "evaluation and treatment." Pt. states that his pain is in the midline lumbar spine, is constant, and occasionally radiates across R buttock to R post thigh to just AK, worse w/ sitting and prolonged standing, better w/ rest, esp. sleeping on L side. No c/o sensory symptoms. Neg. B/B. Meds: Indocin, Tagamet.

O: Alert, cooperative. Does not appear to be in acute distress. X-ray, L spine, Apr. 23, 200x: mild facet DJD, otherwise WNL. GMT NL BLE, FAROM BLE. L spine AROM: FB full, BB 1/2 w/ pain in midline L spine, SB full B. Reflexes 2+/symm. BLE. SLT intact, symm. BLE and L spine. Neg. SLR to 85 degrees B; neg. Fabere B. SIJ screen WNL. Neg. spasm, TTP, deformity, L spine. Posture WNL. Gait WNL.

A: Chronic LBP syndrome; mild L spine DJD; probable lumbar extension dysfunction; r/o HNP.

P: MH today in clinic, F/B prone active extension exercises, 10–15 reps; postural, lifting, and sleeping hints. I/C obtained for Rx. No adverse reaction to Rx noted. Cont. w/ above program in clinic bid X 3–5 days; reevaluate for home program on discharge. Understands all; no questions. Scheduled for back school May 3, 201x.

—**Ron Therapist, PT**

Exhibit 2-A-3 Sample SOAPG Patient Evaluation Note

The following is a physical therapist's initial note for a hospitalized inpatient evaluated in a comprehensive rehabilitation center:

Multidisciplinary Rehabilitation Center, Anytown, USA
May 1, 201x

S: 47 y o M, college math professor, dx: chronic LBP syndrome (Dr. Brown), referred for "evaluation and treatment." Pt. states that his pain is in the midline lumbar spine, is constant, and occasionally radiates across R buttock to R post thigh to just AK, worse w/ sitting and prolonged standing, better w/ rest, esp. sleeping on L side. No c/o sensory symptoms. Neg. B/B. Hx of sx for 1 yr, since fall on ice onto back while shoveling snow at home (Apr. 19, 201x). Spent 10 days in hospital, undergoing lumbar traction, WFE, MH, and US, with initial success. Intermittent OP Rx since then. (Records w/ pt. and reviewed.) No prior back hx, no subsequent injury. Med. hx: AODM, controlled by diet, stomach ulcer, GB surgery, Feb. 1998. Meds: Indocin, Tagamet.

O: Alert, cooperative. Does not appear to be in acute distress. X-ray, L spine, Apr. 23, 201x: mild facet DJD, otherwise WNL. GMT NL BLE, FAROM BLE. L spine AROM: FB full, BB 1/2 w/ pain in midline L spine, SB full B. Reflexes 2+/symm. BLE. SLT intact, symm. BLE and L spine. Neg. SLR to 85 degrees B, neg. Fabere B. SIJ screen WNL. Neg. spasm, TTP, deformity, L spine. Posture WNL. Gait WNL.

A: Chronic LBP syndrome; mild L spine DJD; probable lumbar extension dysfunction; r/o HNP.

P: MH today in clinic, F/B prone active extension exercises, 10–15 reps, postural, lifting, and sleeping hints. I/C obtained for Rx. No adverse reaction to Rx. Cont. w/ above program in clinic bid. X 3–5 days, reevaluate for home program on discharge. Understands all, no questions. Scheduled for back school May 3, 201x.

G: Centralize RLE pain X 3 days, decrease LBP 25% X 3–5 days, RTW sx-free in 1 week, increase back extensor mm strength X 4–6 wks, postural awareness, I ADL w/o sx.

—Ron Therapist, PT

2-B

Examples of Acceptable Techniques for Patient Care Documentation Error Correction

---

Exhibit 2-B-1 Example of Appropriate Patient Treatment Entry Error Correction (lining through material to be deleted and initialing and dating the correction)

Mainline Community Hospital, Mainline, USA
Occupational Therapy Clinic
Dec. 19, 201x/1400

S: 38 y o F, occupation: comic book illustrator, w/ dx of R CTS, s/p CTR (DOS: Dec. 10, 201x). Referred for ROM evaluation and AROM and strengthening program for RUE. P w/o complaints today. R wrist in neutral brace. Meds include Tylenol and Flexeril.

O: Alert, cooperative. GMT deferred. AROM out of brace, R wrist: flex: 65 degrees, ext: 60 degrees, RD: 25 degrees, UD: 25 degrees. SLT intact. Wound, volar wrist fully healed healing/covered with Steri-strips. ~~Negative~~ (R.P.H. 12/19/201x) Slight swelling.

A: Resolving R CTS, s/p R CTR.

P: Teach pt. R wrist AROM as ordered. I/C obtained. Demonstrated understanding of exercises; to do as home program, 10 reps each direction tid. Cold pack p.r.n. before or after exercises. No adverse reaction to Rx. F/U 2–3 wks or p.r.n. earlier.

G: STG: Increase pain-free AROM R wrist to symmetrical w/ L x 2–3 wks.

LTG: I pain-free comic book illustration and other ADL x 1–2 mos, RTW.

—Reginald P. Hasenfus, Jr., OTR/L

Exhibit 2-B-2 Example of Appropriate Patient Care Documentation Entry Error Correction (lining through material to be deleted, initialing and dating the correction, and writing brief justification for correction in margin alongside deletion)

Mainline Community Hospital Mainline, USA
Occupational Therapy Clinic
Dec. 19, 201x/1400

S: 38 y o F, occupation: comic book illustrator, w/ dx of R CTS, s/p CTR (DOS: Dec. 10, 201x). Referred for ROM evaluation and AROM and strengthening program for RUE. Pt. W/o complaints today. R wrist in neutral brace. Meds include Motrin and Indocin.

O: Alert, cooperative. GMT deferred. AROM out of brace, R wrist: flex: 65 degrees, ext: 60 degrees, RD: 25 degrees, UD: 25 degrees. SLT intact. Wound, volar wrist healing/covered with Steri-strips. Negative swelling.

A: Resolving R CTS, s/p R CTR.

P: Teach pt. R wrist AROM as ordered. I/C obtained. Demonstrated understanding of exercises; to do as home program, 10 reps each direction tid. Cold pack p.r.n. before or after exercises. No adverse reaction to Rx. F/U 2–3 wks or p.r.n. earlier.

G: STG: Increase pain-free AROM R wrist to symmetrical w/ L X in 2–3 wks.

LTG: I pain-free comic book illustration and other ADL × 12 mos, RTW.

—**Reginald P. Hasenfus, Jr., OTR/L**

Bitte, Violet P. Pt. 340047899   **O'Boyle, Doree M. Pt. #40048901**
DOB: Mar. 30, 1955   **DOB: May 1, 1967**

R.P.H.
12/19/201x
NOT THIS PATIENT

Exhibit 2-B-3 Example of Personalized Patient Care Documentation for Home Exercise Program

HealthUniversal, P.C.
123 Main Street
Anytown, USA
(210) 555-1212

June 1, 201x

Tom Doe's Home Exercises for Low Back Pain

Do the following exercises every other day for 60 days, to your comfort tolerance (in this order):
After gentle moist heat × 10 minutes (e.g., bath):
Face up: single & double knees to chest × 10;
Hip swaying side to side × 10;
Long sitting (feet extended straight ahead): hamstring stretch: lean forward, no bouncing, one minute hold × 2;
"Indian sitting": gentle stretch, one minute hold × 2;

Face down: press up with stomach sagged (cobra position) × 10.

1. Level surface walking—⅛ to ¼ mile. Try to limit excessive hip motion and arm swing.

2. As an alternative to walking, try exercise bike: 8–15 minutes, no or low resistance, every other session.

3. End with 10 standing back bends with hands on hips.

Good luck with these exercises! Call me with any questions or problems. Have a great start to the summer! I'll see you back in the clinic in two months for your recheck, or earlier, if needed.

Ron Scott, PT

Exhibit 2-B-4 Example of a Telephone Conversation Documentation Form for Inclusion in a Patient's Health Record

HealthUniversal, P.C.
123 Main Street
Anytown, USA
(210) 555-1212

Telephone Conversation Memorandum

Date: _____   Time: _____ AM/PM

Name of Parties Conversing: _____

Parties' phone numbers/contact information: _____

Subject discussed: _____

Notes: _____

Exhibit 2-B-5 Example of Communication of Patient Discharge Between Physical Therapist and Physician

ABC Health, Inc.
321 Side Street
Firstline, TX 78108
(210) 555-6260

DATE: _____
RE: _____

Dear Physician:

The attached discharge summary on your patient is being faxed to you for your records. Please note that this patient is being discharged from physical therapy today.

If you have any questions, concerns, or further orders regarding this patient, please contact us. Thank you for referring this patient to our clinic for care.

Respectfully,

Dr. Ron Scott, PT, EdD
Therapist-in-Charge

CHAPTER 3

The Patient Care Record in Legal Proceedings

This chapter focuses on the patient care record as a business and legal document and examines its uses in administrative and legal proceedings. Spoliation—the intentional alteration or destruction of patient care records—and its consequences are examined. The health professional–patient legal privilege against disclosure of patient care-related information is also explored. The chapter concludes with a discussion of confidentiality issues concerning patient protected health information (PHI), including an example of a HIPAA-correct patient authorization for release of records.

PATIENT CARE RECORDS AS BUSINESS AND LEGAL DOCUMENTS

Chapter 2 addressed the principal purposes for which healthcare professionals document information about patients in patient care records. Although the primary reason for creating and maintaining patient care records is to have a database of clinically pertinent medical information readily available for use by healthcare providers caring for patients now or in the future, many other purposes also exist for the creation of these records. This chapter describes the nature and uses of the patient care record as a business document and a legal document post-HIPAA (Health Insurance Portability and Accountability Act of 1996).

As a business document, the patient care record serves a wide range of administrative functions. These include, among others: serving as the basis for justifying reimbursement for healthcare services from third-party payer entities, creating a database for monitoring quality, establishing appropriate risk management activities, and providing a resource base for research and training.

As a legal document, the patient care record simultaneously serves to protect the legal interests of all participants in the healthcare delivery system, including patients and their families and significant others, healthcare providers and their support staffs, healthcare clinical managers and administrators, and healthcare organizations and systems. In healthcare malpractice litigation, for example, a patient care record can simultaneously be used as a sword by a patient-plaintiff and as a shield by the patient's healthcare provider-defendant.

PATIENT-FOCUSED DOCUMENTATION: THE ROAD MAP TO QUALITY CARE AND EFFECTIVE RISK MANAGEMENT

Despite its broad range of variegated uses as a legal instrument, healthcare recordkeeping is not and should not (with limited exceptions) be carried out with a defensive legal focus. Rather, the creation of patient care records should be guided primarily by patient welfare-oriented healthcare principles. All healthcare professional disciplines and the overwhelming majority of healthcare providers have as their altruistic, narrow focus the welfare of the patients under their care, whom they are attempting to restore to optimal health.

Healthcare professionals documenting entries in patient care records often have little time to ponder carefully over what they write about patients under their care, as such a significant proportion of healthcare delivery occurs under emergency circumstances or under the time constraints of cost-containment-focused managed care. Even so, healthcare professionals are acutely focused on their patients and on recording in an objective manner data that will create a historical basis for the efficacious continuity of care. They rightly are not primarily focused on self-protection from legal action.

In large part because of this focus and the objectivity inherent in healthcare recordkeeping, patient care records have always commanded a high degree of credibility in legal proceedings as important evidence of a patient's health status and of the quality and quantity of patient care. There are several reasons why patient care records enjoy such a high degree of respectability as substantive evidence in administrative and legal proceedings. First, assuming that patient care documentation is performed in a timely manner, it probably represents the most accurate objective evidence of a patient's health status at a given point in time. And second, because healthcare providers document care primarily with the patient's welfare in mind, what they document is largely unbiased.

By analogy, documentation by an attorney of attorney- or attorney agent-generated information about a client's case is called *attorney work product,* which shares many similarities but also has important differences from a healthcare provider's care-related documentation about a patient. Both classes of professional documentation memorialize the professional's assessment of a client's condition or case. Both enjoy qualified immunity (protection) from disclosure to other persons. However, attorney work product does not enjoy the same status as substantive, objective evidence as does patient care documentation.

Attorney work product is, by definition, documentation prepared on a client's behalf in anticipation of litigation. Only by asserting the claim of its potential use in litigation on behalf of a client can attorneys withhold from disclosure to litigation opponents or others the information contained in such documentation. By its very nature, attorney work product documentation is, or at least is deemed to contain, information that is biased in favor of the position advocated on behalf of the client served. Therefore, even if it were not privileged information, attorney work product would not normally qualify in court as substantive evidence of the truth, unlike patient care documentation.

There are serious dangers inherent when healthcare providers adopt a philosophy of defensive, legally oriented patient care documentation. Where patient care documentation has the appearance of having been written primarily to protect or "cover" providers rather than to record objectively patient status or care, its credibility as substantive evidence of patient status and care becomes suspect. Patient care records written in anticipation of litigation do not usually qualify as substantive evidence about the quality of care rendered. Defensive patient care documentation cost $45.6 billion in 2008, according to Michelle Mello of the Harvard School of Public Health.[1]

CREATION AND MAINTENANCE OF PATIENT RECORDS

State and federal statutes, administrative regulations (especially pursuant to the federal HIPAA statute and its implementing regulations), and organization, system, and accreditation entity standards typically establish the parameters of a healthcare provider's or organization's duty to create and maintain patient health records. Even in the absence of such regulatory guidance, however, primary healthcare providers have a common law duty to make and store patient care records. Failure to create a patient care record and maintain it on a patient's behalf for a specified period is a breach of duty owed to that patient. And if the breach of that duty can be tied to some sort of patient injury, then an actionable healthcare malpractice lawsuit for negligent (or intentional) failure to document care or retain records can be successfully pursued by the patient.

How are patient care records stored? Depending on state or federal law, treatment records are stored as originals, on computer disks, hard drives or microfilm, or otherwise. State or federal statutory, regulatory, and common law as well as professional association and institutional practice and accreditation standards control or provide guidance on how long a patient care record must be maintained. Different rules often apply to hospitals, other treatment facilities, and individual healthcare providers. More restrictive rules often apply to special situations, such as infants', children's, and cancer patient records. Under many state statutory laws, for example, minors' health records must be preserved until some number of years after the minor patients reach the age of 18 years, the legal age of majority.

Irrespective of any legal patient care record retention requirements, providers and facilities should customarily and routinely keep patients' records at least until the applicable statute of limitations, or "time clock" for bringing legal actions incident to care, has expired. Remember, when considering the lengths of various statutes of limitations, that different "time clocks" apply to actions brought by patients under tort (wrong-based) theories of healthcare malpractice and other potential bases of liability, such as breach of contract, fraud, and criminal law violations (in which statutes of limitations are usually longer).

Some authorities recommend that providers maintain patient records containing significant data until after the deaths of such patients.[2] In addition to the legal requirements for retaining critical patient information, providers may be ethically responsible for preserving this kind of data about their patients to ensure continuity of care. Even for routine information, it may be prudent to retain patient care records for 7 to 10 years, irrespective of whether state or federal law allows for their earlier destruction. This is sound advice even in a case in which the provider has disengaged from care for a particular patient.

NONAVAILABILITY OF PATIENT CARE RECORDS AS EVIDENCE OF SPOLIATION

The adverse consequences when healthcare providers fail to maintain patient care records as prescribed by law, practice standards, or custom are potentially severe. In particular, courts adjudicating healthcare malpractice cases in which records are unavailable for patients' (and providers') use may permit juries to infer or even presume[3] healthcare malpractice against providers under the theory of spoliation of records.

Spoliation is a legal term of art that describes the intentional destruction or material alteration of a document by a party for the purpose of changing or concealing its original meaning. (Courts normally disallow a patient legal cause of action against a provider or healthcare organization for negligent, or unintentional, spoliation.[4]) A charge of spoliation of patient treatment records can give rise to civil, criminal, and adverse administrative and professional association actions against a healthcare provider. As a criminal matter, spoliation can be both a form of fraud and obstruction of justice. If it is planned, discussed, and/or carried out in concert by two or more healthcare providers, spoliation of a patient care record may also give rise to a civil or criminal action for conspiracy. (*Conspiracy* involves a situation in which two or more people agree to commit an unlawful act. When charged as a criminal action, it is a separate offense from any underlying crime, such as fraud, obstruction of justice, or perjury.)

Also, the wrongful intentional alteration of patient care records with an intent to deceive is a violation of most, if not all, healthcare professional ethics codes. A charge of spoliation can result in adverse licensure action, such as suspension or revocation, and imposition of a monetary fine by the provider's state licensing board, and of reporting of the adverse licensure and/or credentialing action to the National Practitioner Data Bank.[5]

Spoliation of patient care documentation is the intentional destruction or material alteration of an entry for the purpose of changing or concealing its original meaning.

Spoliation of patient care records can be considered as the civil healthcare analog to the criminal law concept of *obstruction of justice*. The healthcare provider who intentionally alters or destroys records "obstructs" the effective delivery of patient care by distorting the true account of a patient's course of care.

Healthcare providers can commit spoliation of patient care records even when they do not have any malicious intent to defraud anyone—patients, their attorneys, legal authorities, or others. For example, consider the hypothetical case in which a patient lodges a complaint against a healthcare facility, alleging poor quality of care and a resultant adverse outcome. The patient's letter to the facility triggers the flagging of the patient's record and designation of the patient's care as a potentially compensable event.

Now assume that the healthcare clinicians named in the claim as parties responsible for the patient's care are asked by the facility's administrator to review the patient's record, without being told that the patient was dissatisfied with care. In this hypothetical situation, assume that some providers mistakenly presume that they are being asked to review the record for quality self-assessment.

If the providers see documentation entries that are obviously erroneous or incomplete, they may be inclined or tempted to "correct" the record by adding information without annotating the supplemental material as a new entry or by removing original material and substituting new entries. This is especially tempting when there are blank lines in the original notation or when individual patient care entries are written on separate pages.

This tendency to "correct" patient care documentation entries in hindsight may be a natural instinct, in large part reflective of healthcare providers' innate concern for ensuring accuracy and clarity in patient care documentation. As was emphasized in Chapter 2, such considerations reflect the principal purpose for patient care documentation (i.e., effective communication of pertinent clinical information to others having a need to know).

Assume hypothetically that a treatment entry seemingly requiring clarification appears as follows:

May 3, 201x

P: Status post right proximal humeral fracture, nondisplaced, Apr. 15, 201x.

S: Neurovascular intact. Minimal swelling and c/o pain. In sling, with arm adducted and internally rotated, held against abdomen. Med: Tylenol 3.

P: To PT for ROM. Follow-up 2 wks or p.r.n.

G: Promote healing, prevent adhesive capsulitis X 4–6 wks, independent ADL.

—J. Ortho, MD

The above note, when reviewed by Dr. Ortho, might be "corrected" to read as follows, with substitution of a new page containing the amended entry in place of the original one:

May 3, 201x

P: Status post right proximal humeral fracture, nondisplaced, Apr. 15, 201x.

S: *Doing very well.* Neurovascular intact. Minimal swelling and minimal c/o pain. In sling, with arm adducted and internally rotated, and held against abdomen. Med: *Tylenol.*

P: To PT *within 72 hrs* for passive and active assist ROM to pain tolerance only. Follow-up 2 wks or p.r.n.

G: Promote healing, prevent adhesive capsulitis X 4–6 wks; independent ADL.

—J. Ortho, MD

The changes, although arguably only minor in nature, make the record appear as if more findings were observed and more detailed orders made than originally appeared. In this case, Dr. Ortho actually believed that he recalled hearing the patient say that she was doing "very well." He also remembered telephoning physical therapy to ask the therapist to examine the patient within 72 hours of referral and to carry out only passive and active assist range of motion with the patient. He just forgot to annotate those items the first time around. Imagine the impression on a judge or jury if the provider in the hypothetical case were on the stand in a health-care malpractice trial trying to explain his substituted progress note after the original had been located. Even if the physical therapist corroborated what Dr. Ortho wrote the second time around, the judge might still direct the jury to presume negligence based on spoliation of patient care records.

Healthcare professionals and administrative employees of healthcare organizations are not at liberty to alter existing patient care documentation notation, even for the innocent purpose of clarifying an ambiguous or incomplete prior entry. Even though the hypothetical alteration noted previously was performed without any wrongful intent, it would probably be characterized as such by the patient's attorney and might be so construed by the court if the potentially compensable event (PCE) were to ripen into a healthcare malpractice legal action.

If the surgeon in this case forgot to annotate some crucial clinical information that needed to be added to the patient record, then the surgeon should have added the missing information by way of a new entry explaining the prior omission. Such a proper new entry might appear as follows:

May 4, 201x

P: Status post right proximal humeral fracture, nondisplaced, Apr. 15, 201x.

S: Regarding my earlier note of May 3, 201x, the following examination and follow-up information is added: The patient reported that she was doing "very well" on exam. I coordinated telephonically with physical therapy for her to be seen within 72 hrs for passive and active assist ROM to pain tolerance only. The patient's medication was Tylenol vs. Tylenol 3.

G: Promote healing; prevent adhesive capsulitis X 4–6 wks; independent ADL.

—J. Ortho, MD

Because of this natural propensity on the part of providers to correct inaccurate patient care record information—whether for self-serving reasons, out of concern for patients, or for accuracy—organization/system administrators and risk managers should not routinely permit providers, consultants, or others to review original patient care records involving known PCEs. For the protection of patients, providers, and the organization or system, interested parties should only be given clear, complete photocopies of patient care records to review. In a legal case involving a purportedly lost patient care record entry, the facility administrator and/ or risk manager might even be held legally accountable if the original records were in their possession at the time of probable loss.

Unfortunately, unlike the hypothetical case presented above, most spoliation of patient care records probably is not performed unknowingly or innocently. In fact, health law and other authorities express concern that spoliation of health records may be a growing problem. One authority, Dr. Robert Prosser, attributes the increase in the incidence in patient treatment record spoliation during the past five years to a defensive reaction by healthcare providers to the fear of healthcare malpractice litigation and liability. Dr. Prosser correctly noted in his article that most clinicians who alter patient treatment entries are competent, well-meaning providers who inadvertently document their good patient care inadequately and often "correct" entries without any intent to deceive.[6]

Clinic, department, and risk managers, and organization/system administrators should educate all clinicians who write in patient records about spoliation and its consequences and, in particular, should emphasize that it is wrong and legally indefensible—irrespective of the motive for doing it. Spoliation of a patient care record is a shortcut to certain settlement of a healthcare malpractice case, usually on terms unfavorable to healthcare providers and organizations. Along with such a settlement come the adverse personal consequences to individual providers discussed in Chapter 2, including the possible inclusion of providers' names in the National Practitioner Data Bank. A settlement under these circumstances that would otherwise have been unnecessary is also detrimental to the reputation of the healthcare organization in the community, adversely affecting its business interests.

Once it is concluded that alteration, destruction, or even negligent loss of patient care records that are under the control of healthcare providers individually, or the healthcare facility generally, has taken place, there is good reason to settle a healthcare malpractice case, rather than go to court. This is so even in the face of clearly disputable patient allegations, because of the danger that the court will allow an inference or presumption of negligence and the possibility of a punitive damages award in the event of a finding of liability. Because of these considerations, most insurers of healthcare professionals settle such cases.

Investigators and document examiners have little trouble spotting patient care entries that have been altered or supplemented without creating a new dated entry. They often need only examine the original records with the naked eye to see signs of alteration. Such signs may include the following:

- Differences in handwriting style within an entry, including different slanting of added words or individual alphabetical letters, and mixed cursive and printing handwriting styles
- Use of different writing instruments within an entry
- Obvious erasures and other forms of obliteration, such as the use of correction liquid or permanent marker
- Nonuniform crowding of words, phrases, or symbols within an entry, especially between lines or in the margins of the entry

Signs of substitution of rewritten patient care entries, although often more difficult to detect, may include the following:

- Differences in paper type or quality in the substituted entry and the record generally
- Graphemic (letter) differences in entries (e.g., pressure, slant, and spacing of letters)
- Stylistic differences in entries (e.g., longer, more detailed note on day of incident in issue)
- Binder holes or other markings that do not match up with the rest of the record
- Date and/or time discrepancies
- Subsequent entries (by the provider committing spoliation of records or by other providers) that are incongruous or confusing, based on material contained in the substituted entry
- Observations or findings in the substituted entry that could not have been observed or known at the purported time of notation
- Handwriting style and/or quality of documentation that is inconsistent with documentation exemplars of the writer

For more subtle alterations, document examiners rely on sophisticated scientific detection instruments and techniques. These include, among many others, ultraviolet and infrared light analysis, spectrometry and chromatography, chemical analysis of ink used in treatment entries, fingerprint analysis, and computer data retrieval methods.

The foundation for establishing spoliation in court requires the patient-plaintiff's attorney to establish that the defendant-healthcare providers and organization had a legal duty to preserve and safeguard any patient care records in question.[7] Once it is established that the defendant(s) wrong-fully disposed of patient records in issue, "all things are presumed against the wrongdoer."[8] The simple lesson is, don't alter or dispose of patient care documentation in any form that may be needed as evidence in potential litigation.

DEFENDING AGAINST AN INFERENCE OR PRESUMPTION OF NEGLIGENCE

When a court in a malpractice case rules as a matter of law that the jury either can infer or must presume negligence against a provider or health-care facility based on lost or altered patient care records, the defense attorney normally has the special burden to either dispel the inference or rebut the presumption to prevent imposition of liability. In particular, to rebut a presumption of negligence based on spoliation, the defense must introduce some evidence that negates the presumption that providers or the facility was responsible for the loss of patient records.

What types of evidence might be sufficient to dispel a presumption of spoliation? At the simplest (or perhaps most complex) level, a provider accused of spoliation can testify convincingly that he or she did not alter or destroy patient record entries. The defense can introduce investigators, document examiners, and other scientific expert witnesses during its own case to testify that spoliation did not occur. The defense can also intro-duce doubt about the source of clear spoliation into the jury's mind if it can show that the patient-plaintiff possessed or controlled his or her own records during the pendency of the legal process.

Once a healthcare provider's defense attorney produces solid credible evidence negating a presumption of alteration or destruction of patient records at the hands of the provider, any presumption of negligence based upon spoliation is normally dispelled, and the patient-plaintiff's full bur-den of proving malpractice to prevail is restored.

SEGREGATION OF LITIGATION PATIENT CARE RECORDS

In large part because of the dangers of spoliation either at the hands of healthcare providers, patients, or others, facility risk managers should routinely segregate original patient records and other tangible items such as imaging studies, photographs, electronic monitoring tapes, microscopic slides, and tissue samples involving PCEs and secure them to prevent their unauthorized removal. Release of health records or information should be handled centrally by the facility risk manager or health records administrator. Requests for records involving PCEs should be coordinated with the facility's legal counsel before release.

OWNERSHIP OF PATIENT CARE RECORDS

What entity owns patient health records: the healthcare organization, individual healthcare providers, or patients? Or do all of them co-own patient records? Under early common law, before state and federal statutory law controlled this area of law, physicians and hospitals had absolute ownership rights to records of patients under their care. Under this scheme, the patients had no legal right of access to information contained in their records and little or no legal recourse if record access was denied to them.

Under modern patient record statutes, healthcare providers creating the records still own the physical records. Before April 14, 2003, when compliance with HIPAA privacy regulations was first in effect, in most states, patients had either direct or indirect access to the information contained in their healthcare records. Some of the reasons offered by authorities for favoring ready patient access to health records include the following:

- It fosters a closer provider–patient relationship, particularly when there is also good communication generally between health professional and patient.
- Under consumerism principles, the patient has the right to rebut and compel correction of false or inaccurate information contained in his or her patient care record. False information in patient care records can form the basis for denial of health insurance or even employment, if physical performance standards are legitimate requisites to employment. False information can also form the basis for a legal action against the provider or healthcare organization for defamation or intentional infliction of emotional distress.
- A trend in healthcare law philosophy holds that, although the healthcare provider may own the physical record of a patient, the patient has proprietary rights to the sensitive information contained

in it, because such information is personal to the patient and the patient has an autonomous right to it.

Before HIPAA, 28 states, by statute, already gave patients full access to information contained in their patient care records that were in the possession of individual healthcare providers and hospitals (excluding mental health records, or cases where information released might endanger the patient or another person). Patients whose health records were maintained in federal healthcare facilities also generally had the same right of access to information contained in their records.

In states where direct patient access to healthcare information was restricted, administrative hurdles to be overcome by patients to gain access to their records included the following: the requirement for a court order before release of records, release only for potentially compensable events or to an attorney, release to the patient only after demonstration of "good cause," and substitution of a report or summary of care in lieu of actual patient care records, at healthcare providers' and organizations' discretion.[9]

After April 14, 2003, patients nationwide became entitled under HIPAA to copies of their PHI upon signed written request. Under federal HIPAA regulations, copies must normally be given to patients within 30 days (up to 60 days for good cause). Patients can be compelled to pay reasonable copying and mailing costs for their records. Patients also have the right to have erroneous PHI corrected by a provider or facility, and/or their disagreement with information annotated, within 60 to 90 days of notice.[10]

In some healthcare systems, patients retain their own patient care records, under what is called an "ambulatory record system." Such a system of patient care record maintenance may offer important advantages in this era of managed care and cost-containment, including ready access to the records by healthcare providers caring for the patient, enhancement of patient self-awareness and education about personal health status, and decreased cost for record storage by healthcare organizations.

Disadvantages also exist in an ambulatory patient care record system, however. These include the danger of spoliation of record entries by patients or their representatives; emotional distress associated with patients reading about, but perhaps not adequately understanding, their health status; and the possibility that patients will have a greater propensity to bring claims or lawsuits based on perceived healthcare malpractice.

From a patient's perspective, the most effective way to gain release of the patient's own records is to make the request in writing. Oral requests may carry less weight. Also, insist on copies of the actual records, rather than a provider's own summary of the information contained therein.

What about ownership of patient care records after dissolution of a clinical practice group or the retirement or death of the custodial healthcare provider? When a clinical practice dissolves, providers have an ethical and legal obligation to notify their patients of the dissolution and request that the patients provide the retiring providers with the names of substitute healthcare professionals to whom copies of the patients' records will be forwarded. Original records should be retained by the original healthcare providers, where allowed by law, at least until the expiration of applicable statutes of limitations for healthcare malpractice legal actions. (Note that Texas, for example, requires retention of PHI for a minimum of seven years after the last date that care was rendered to a patient.[11])

When a primary healthcare provider dies, the patient care records in that provider's possession normally become the property of the deceased professional's estate. The executor or administrator of the estate—a "business associate" under HIPAA regulations[12]—must then advertise the availability of copies of the patients' records for transfer to other healthcare providers. Creditors of the deceased provider may also claim a right to payment of patient bills owed to the provider before his or her death.

HOW TO HANDLE A PATIENT REQUEST FOR RELEASE OF PATIENT CARE RECORD INFORMATION

There are many reasons other than seeking a legal review for suspected healthcare malpractice for which a patient may request his or her health records from a provider or facility. The patient may be transferring to another geographical area of the country or world, or the provider may be moving or retiring from practice and the patient is responding to the provider's request to have records transferred. Nevertheless, patients often request their records to take them to attorneys for legal review for suspected malpractice.

As was explained previously, federal law requires providers to release PHI to patients on request. A prudent patient relations and risk-management measure is to also have a healthcare provider or small group of providers request a meeting with the patient to give the patient an opportunity to ask questions about his or her health status or care and have them answered in straightforward, layperson's language by their providers. This form of communication and show of concern may prevent a lawsuit. Such an offer should first be coordinated with the facility risk manager and perhaps with legal counsel to avoid violating the attorney–client privilege in the event that the patient is already represented by legal counsel.

When meeting with a disgruntled patient under such circumstances, providers must exercise caution not to use jargon in speaking to the patient and his or her family/significant others. Rather, they should break down information into simple layperson's English (or Spanish, Vietnamese, and so on, as appropriate, with or without an interpreter).

This sort of meeting between provider(s) and patient may be the last best chance to prevent a claim or litigation over perceived substandard care, so it is vital that providers know how to conduct themselves in such circumstances. Facility providers and support staff should attend in-service education on communication skills with patients and perhaps should conduct mock exercises on how to deal effectively with disgruntled patients. This training is the responsibility of the facility risk manager or outside risk management consultant, as appropriate. Managed care and its inherent time constraints make the scheduling of such meetings between providers and patients more difficult. They should, however, be undertaken, because providers are *fiduciaries* (i.e., in a position of special trust, charged to place patient interests above their own) for their patients and because it is in providers' and healthcare organizations' own best interests.

Ask yourself whether the typical patient would understand the following explanation of his or her diagnosis: "The MRI and electromyographic studies reveal, and my neuromusculoskeletal clinical examination confirms, that you display increased polyphasic potentials in the musculature supplied by your right common peroneal nerve and have point tenderness to palpation over the tibial plateau. My diagnosis, therefore, is rule out intercortical lesion of the right knee secondary to trauma, with peroneal nerve compression." Probably not!

Just as lawyers learn (or should learn) through continuing legal education courses to break out of "legalese" when speaking to clients, healthcare professionals must learn to break down health jargon into layperson's language for their patients and their significant others. The esoteric explanation expounded by the surgeon above should have been stated as follows to the patient: "You had a bad fall. I believe you may have broken your right knee. You may also have some nerve damage involving muscles in your right shin and foot."

Studies have revealed that patients often do not understand even the terms that most healthcare providers would consider elemental, such as "hypertension," "oral," and "asymptomatic." The failure to communicate clinical information effectively to patients probably leads to disgruntled patients and healthcare malpractice legal actions more often than explaining terms and parameters of patient examinations, evaluative findings, diagnoses, prognoses, and intervention instructions in simple language at patients' levels of comprehension, and soliciting and answering patient and family/significant other questions effectively.

The final point regarding release of patient records concerns copying fees. HIPAA and most state statutes permit healthcare providers and facilities to charge a reasonable statutory fee for copying records and, in many cases, also a reasonable mailing fee. Providers and health records administrators should exercise prudence when setting such fees to prevent already angry patients from becoming even more so. Such anger might just be vented by the patient through filing a healthcare malpractice lawsuit. Courts, too, closely scrutinize the propriety of health records copying fees.

ADMISSION OF THE PATIENT CARE RECORD IN COURT AS EVIDENCE

Patient care records serve a myriad of functions in legal proceedings in both the pretrial and trial stages of civil and criminal proceedings. In criminal prosecutions, patient records may be used to aid police investigations, determine the extent of injuries or cause of death of a victim, and establish a defendant's competency to stand trial or sanity, among other things. In civil proceedings other than those involving healthcare malpractice, health records are vital to the administration of justice as well. In motor vehicle or other accident cases, and in workers' compensation actions, patient care records are introduced to establish the extent of a party's injuries or disability, to ascertain a party's functional or work capacity, and to justify a plaintiff 's request for damages based on the quantity and cost of healthcare rendered, among other uses.

In healthcare malpractice cases, patient care records are used as discussed above to prove or disprove patient injury from healthcare provider or organization malpractice, and to establish monetary losses, or "damages." They also are often introduced as substantive evidence of a patient-plaintiff's health status and to evaluate the quantity and quality of care rendered to a patient.

Patient care records typically are requested by a patient or the patient's attorney long before a potentially compensable event ripens into a lawsuit. In states where a court order is required to release treatment records to patients, their attorneys may have to seek a court order and "discover" the records from the official custodian of the records through issuance of a legal document called a *subpoena duces tecum*. A *subpoena duces tecum* is an order to the custodian of documents or other physical things that are pertinent to issues in a legal controversy to deliver them to a particular place, such as a copying center, or to bring them when testifying at a legal proceeding, such as a pretrial deposition or a trial.[13]

Patients whose records are subpoenaed have statutory rights of challenge to subpoena of their health records. The subpoenaing party must normally send the patient a *notice of subpoena* and send the healthcare provider having custody over the records a *certificate of compliance*. This certificate is a sworn statement made by the subpoenaing party to the record custodian that the patient received the notice of subpoena. Normally, the record custodian must wait a statutory period, for example, 15 days, before forwarding the records to the party with the subpoena, to give the patient sufficient time to mount a challenge to the order to produce, if so desired. In a Rhode Island reported legal case, the state Supreme Court held that patients whose records are subpoenaed before investigative grand juries also have the right to notice and challenge of the subpoena.[14]

Subpoena duces tecum: A court order to the custodian of patient treatment records that are pertinent to issues in a legal case to deliver them to a business location or to bring them when testifying at a legal proceeding, such as a pretrial deposition or a trial.

When used at trial as substantive evidence of patient status or care, a patient care record is hearsay evidence. *Hearsay* evidence is any statement (oral, written, or otherwise) made outside of the setting of a trial offered at trial as substantive evidence of the truth of the matter asserted in that statement. Under the "hearsay rule," absent some recognized exception, hearsay evidence is inadmissible in a court of law.

That does not mean that evidence that would otherwise be excludable hearsay cannot be used for purposes other than offering it for its truth. For example, a written hearsay statement might properly be shown to a witness testifying at trial, whose memory is weak, to refresh the witness's present recollection of an event, without admitting the document into evidence. This use of hearsay evidence is called *present recollection refreshed*. A witness is better prepared to answer attorneys' questions and makes a better impression on a judge or jury if the witness prepares for deposition or trial in advance by reviewing pertinent records and other documents that will or may be referenced during such testimony.

In addition, what otherwise would be hearsay evidence may be used on cross-examination (after a witness has testified on direct examination) to impeach the witness by showing that the evidence contradicts the witness's in-court testimony. Hearsay evidence contained in patient treatment records may also be used as the basis or foundation of an expert witness's opinion on an issue in controversy.

> **Hearsay** evidence includes any statement (oral, written, or otherwise) made outside of the setting of a trial, offered at trial as substantive evidence of the truth of the matter asserted in that statement. Under the "hearsay rule," absent some recognized exception, hearsay evidence is inadmissible in a court of law.

THE PATIENT CARE RECORD AS A BUSINESS DOCUMENT

When patient care records are offered in a healthcare malpractice trial as hearsay evidence of the truth asserted in them, they are admissible because they are business records, or "records of regularly conducted activity." Under an exception to the hearsay rule,[15] business records are generally admissible as substantive evidence so long as the following four requirements (which may vary from state to state, and in the federal system) are met:

1. The entries in the record are routinely made as part of a "regular course of business."

2. It is part of the regular practice of the business to make such entries.

3. The entries in the records are made contemporaneously with the events recorded.

4. The custodian of the record testifies and swears or affirms that all the preceding requirements apply to the record offered as evidence and "authenticates" the record, making it admissible as evidence.

Patient care records normally meet all the preceding requirements. Before their admission into evidence, the facility health records administrator or another qualified witness testifies to the following:

1. Patient care records are required to be routinely produced in the "regular course" of healthcare delivery by law, accreditation standards, and custom.

2. Patient care entries in health records are customarily made at or near the time of examination or intervention by providers privileged to write in patient records.

3. Patient care records under the custodian's control are protected from unauthorized handling and alteration.

4. The patient care record in issue was not produced in anticipation of litigation.

The custodian of the records must also attest to the authenticity of the records in issue, as is usually evidenced by an authentication page bearing the custodian's signature and stamp. An example of an authentication page is in Exhibit 3–1.

Exhibit 3–1 Example of Authentication of Patient Care Records

[Hospital Letterhead] Patient Records Division
AFFIDAVIT

State of : _____.

County/Parish of : _____ .

Before me, the undersigned authority, personally appeared Mr./Ms. who, being duly sworn, certified as follows:

My name is _____. I am over age twenty-one, am of sound mind, capable of making the following declaration, and personally acquainted with the facts stated herein:

I am the Health Records Administrator of ABC General Hospital and the custodian of all patient care records for the facility. Attached to this affidavit are (#) pages of the clinical record on (patient's full name) from ABC General Hospital. These said pages of records are kept by ABC General Hospital in the regular course of business of the facility for an employee, representative, or physician privileged to practice in ABC General Hospital, with personal knowledge of the events and conditions herein recorded. The entries made in this record were made at or near the time of the events described, or reasonably soon thereafter, and were not transcribed into the record in the anticipation of litigation. The records attached hereto are exact duplicate photocopies of the original. It is a rule of ABC General Hospital not to permit original records to leave the facility.

Patient (full name) has expressly authorized the release of these records in writing (Authorization attached). ABC's legal counsel has determined their release to be in compliance with HIPAA (Health Insurance Portability and Accountability Act of 1996) and subsequent federal regulations.

Sworn and subscribed before me on the _____ day of _____, 201__.

Notary Public for the State of _____. My commission expires _____.

Normally, the "best evidence rule" requires that the custodian produce the original patient care record in court. Under federal evidence rules, and similar rules in most states, an authenticated photocopy is acceptable "secondary" evidence in lieu of the original record, so long as the custodian's explanation of the original's absence satisfies the court as to the trustworthiness of the record copy.

HEALTHCARE PROFESSIONAL–PATIENT LEGAL PRIVILEGES AGAINST BREACH OF CONFIDENTIALITY

The healthcare professional–patient privilege is a testimonial privilege that sometimes precludes the admission of patient care information into evidence in legal proceedings. This evidentiary privilege protecting confidentiality in court is different from the health professional's general duties of confidentiality and fidelity owed to a patient, which are examined separately in the next section of this chapter.

Under early common law, the legal system took a utilitarian approach to claims for testimonial privileges. Only those that met the following four requirements were allowed:

1. The communication originates in confidence.

2. Confidence is essential to the relationship in issue.

3. The relationship merits confidentiality.

4. The harm that would result from disclosure of the confidential communication outweighs the benefit of preserving it.

No healthcare professional–patient privilege was recognized in common law.

Today, most states and the federal system authorize by statute at least physician–patient and mental health professional–patient privileges. Others authorize evidentiary privileges for other healthcare professionals.

There are qualifications to any healthcare professional–patient privilege. It belongs to the patient and not to the healthcare provider. The privilege only applies in situations in which the patient consulted with the provider for care or for a relevant diagnosis in anticipation of intervention. It may not apply in other situations, for example, in which a patient undergoes a functional-capacity evaluation pursuant to a court order or in which a healthcare professional is consulted by the patient (and not by the patient's attorney) for testimony as an expert at trial. The privilege also may not normally apply in administrative workers' compensation actions as to injuries that are at issue in the proceedings. (Note that even in situations in which a testimonial privilege is inapplicable or waived, a treating healthcare provider still has an ethical and legal [depending on state law] obligation to obtain patient consent before releasing patient care records.)

The healthcare professional–patient privilege is subject to many exceptions. Of importance to health professionals is the exception that applies to cases in which a patient's physical or mental condition is in issue in a legal case, such as in motor vehicle or other accident cases.

For healthcare malpractice lawsuits, waiver of the privilege also applies, so that healthcare professionals who are defendants cannot be prevented from testifying about the patient-plaintiff 's condition or care. Under such circumstances, the patient is deemed to have waived the privilege by bringing suit.

CONFIDENTIALITY OF PATIENT CARE INFORMATION

For more than 2000 years, physicians, on entering the practice of medicine, have recited the Hippocratic Oath, which reads as follows:

> You do solemnly swear, each man (or woman)* by whatever he (or she)* holds most sacred that you will be loyal to the Profession of Medicine and just and generous to its members;
>
> That you will lead your lives and practice your art in uprightness and honor;
>
> That into whatever house you shall enter, it shall be for the good of the sick to the utmost of your power, your holding yourselves far aloof from wrong, from corruption, from the tempting of others to vice;
>
> That you will exercise your art solely for the cure of your patients, and will give no drug, perform no operation, for a criminal purpose, even if solicited, far less suggest it;
>
> *That whatsoever you shall see or hear of the lives of men (or women)* which is not fitting to be spoken, you will keep inviolably secret* [emphasis added];
>
> These things do you swear. Let each man (and woman)* bow the head in sign of acquiescence;
>
> And now, if you will be true to this, your oath, may prosperity and good repute be ever yours; the opposite, if you shall prove yourselves forsworn.
>
> [*Author's additions]

Hippocrates recognized, as have scholars, ethicists, and healthcare professionals generally throughout the ages, that a sense of trust in the healthcare provider on the part of a patient concerning the safeguarding of confidential information is crucial to the success of the professional–patient relationship. The duty of confidentiality is what promotes a patient to "open up" to physicians and other healthcare professionals and reveal innermost secrets that must be disclosed to the provider for accurate diagnosis and efficacious intervention for disease and injury.

According to the philosopher Sissela Bok, author of the book *Lying: Moral Choice in Public and Private Life*, four fundamental ethical principles form the foundation for confidentiality inherent in the healthcare professional–patient relationship. These include respect for (1) patient autonomy over information pertaining to that individual, (2) interpersonal relationships and the individual patient's right to confide in a professional of choice, (3) the solemnity of a pledge of confidentiality, and (4) the use of the healthcare professional–patient confidential relationship in meeting compelling societal health needs.[16]

Since the inception of the Hippocratic Oath, all healthcare disciplines and professionals have come to share the same ethical and legal obligation to safeguard confidential information provided to them by their patients. Modernly, the legal duty of health professionals to respect patient confidentiality derives from statutory and common law, administrative (licensure and certification) regulations, and professional association ethics standards.

Also within the scope of patient confidentiality is a patient's constitutional right of privacy regarding issues ranging from the use of contraceptives[17] to terminating a pregnancy.[18] Physicians and nurse practitioners figure prominently in advising patients contemplating such decisions. In these situations, patients frequently turn to their physicians and nurse practitioners for professional advice and information. The provider's advice to the patient enjoys the same degree of constitutional protection as does the patient's right to seek such advice to make an informed, intelligent decision. Regarding confidentiality, abortion is perhaps the most divisive issue facing America (and many other nations) today. More and more, Congress and state legislatures are narrowing a patient's right to choose to terminate a pregnancy, often through statutes that restrict the kind of information that physicians and other primary healthcare providers can impart to women seeking their advice.

Special confidentiality rules are in effect in many or most states for such issues as a patient's HIV status and documentation involving treatment for drug (including alcohol) abuse, venereal disease, and birth control and abortion advice. Special reporting requirements to state agencies also exist in many jurisdictions for conditions such as HIV/AIDS, other venereal diseases, tuberculosis, and for suspected child, spouse, or elder abuse. These reporting requirements supersede patients' rights to confidentiality concerning information of "compelling state interest."

Other exceptions to the requirement for confidentiality of patient information include requests for patient information from law enforcement agencies and discretionary release of information disclosed by patients to providers where patient's conduct poses an imminent threat of death or serious bodily harm to a third party[19] or national security. Many health professional association codes of ethics also address these exceptions.

When a healthcare provider breaches the duty of confidentiality owed to a patient, the patient may have a legal cause of action under federal and state confidentiality statutes. Penalties for violations typically include a civil or administrative monetary fine. Criminal action brought by a state or federal prosecutor is also possible. Disciplinary action under licensing statutes and regulations also is a potential sanction for unauthorized disclosure of a patient's confidences, as is action before a professional association of which the provider is a member for a breach of ethics.

HIPAA imposes administrative, civil, and criminal penalties for wrongful releases of PHI, including a maximum criminal monetary fine of up to $250,000 per Privacy Rule violation, plus up to ten years imprisonment. Civil complaints, submitted in a signed writing, are adjudicated by the Office of Civil Rights (OCR). Criminal actions are prosecuted by the United States Department of Justice.[20]

When no statutory or regulatory remedy exists for violating a patient's confidence, the patient may bring a civil lawsuit against a provider under the common law principle of *invasion of privacy*. There are four recognized classes of invasion of privacy as follows:

1. Unreasonable intrusion on a patient's solitude

2. Unauthorized publicity that portrays a patient in a false light in the public eye

3. Appropriation (use) of a patient's name or characteristics without consent

4. Unauthorized public revelation of private facts about a patient

The aspect of invasion of privacy most often associated with misuse of patient care documentation is the one concerning the public disclosure of private patient facts. Unauthorized disclosure of private patient information, whether done verbally or through the transfer of written documents, is an actionable breach of a healthcare provider's duty of confidentiality.

A patient who successfully sues a provider for invasion of privacy may be awarded damages for emotional and psychological harm as well as physical harm suffered. The patient may also win punitive damages if the violation is egregious.

> HIPAA requires signed written patient authorization for release of PHI for most purposes.

How do private entities gain the right of access to confidential information contained in patient care records? We as people and patients routinely give up our right of confidentiality every time we sign "routine" waivers of confidentiality in the form of patient care record data releases when receiving care, when applying for life or health insurance, when processing healthcare claims, or for a myriad of other seemingly good reasons. An example of a patient care record release appears in Exhibit 3–2.

Exhibit 3–2 Example of a HIPAA-Compliant Patient Authorization for Release of Patient Care Records

ABC HEALTH CARE CLINIC
ANYTOWN, USA

AUTHORIZATION TO RELEASE PATIENT PROTECTED HEALTH INFORMATION (PHI)

I authorize ABC Health Care Clinic, Anytown, USA, to release patient protected health information (PHI) from the medical record of:
Patient Name _____ Date of Birth _____
Inclusive dates for record release _____
Disclose the PHI delineated below to: _____
Address: _____
For the express purpose of: _____
This authorization includes the following, as applicable:
__History & Physical Exams __Diagnosis & Plan of Care

_Medication Lists _Allergy List _Progress Notes_Discharge Summaries
_Diagnostic Imaging Reports _X-Ray/CT/MRI films
_Laboratory Studies _EKG/EEG Reports _EKG/EEG strips
_Immunization Record _Genetic Testing Information
_Other (Specify): _____

I understand that the PHI in my health record may include information relating to sexually transmitted diseases (STDs), including human immunodeficiency virus (HIV) and/or acquired immunodeficiency syndrome (AIDS); mental health services; and treatment for chemical substance abuse.
_I specifically also consent to the release of this information.
_I do not consent to the release of this information.

Any use, other than for the express purpose above, of this PHI without the written consent of the patient, or patient's legal representative, is prohibited.

This authorization request is voluntary. It is independent of any authorization for, or right to, treatment at ABC. I have the legal right to revoke this authorization at any time. Any such revocation must be in the form of a signed writing. Such revocation cannot apply to information already released pursuant to the prior authorization. Unless otherwise revoked, this authorization will expire on the following date, event, or condition: (if none, so state) _____.

In the absence of a specific expiration date, event, or condition, this authorization will expire in 90 days from its signing.

I acknowledge my right to inspect or copy the PHI to be used or disclosed, persuant to the Code of Federal Regulations Section 164.524. I also acknowledge that any disclosure of PHI creates the possibility of unauthorized follow-on disclosure by others. While ABC requires its business associates to comply with the Health Insurance Portability and Accountability Act's (HIPAA's) Privacy Rule, ABC cannot guarantee compliance.

Please contact _____, ABC HIPAA Privacy Officer, with any questions, comments or concerns about this authorization and/or your care at ABC. Thank you.

Signature of patient or legal representative (state relationship, if signed by a legal representative) — Date

Signature of Witness

Consumer advocates urge all individuals to take several steps to ensure that any information on file about them is accurate. First, consumers should inquire of such agencies about any information they might have on them and request a summary of that information. If it is erroneous, as it sometimes is, consumers should take steps to have the data corrected to prevent denial of employment, insurance, or other rights and benefits. Second, consumers should consider "tailoring" any releases they authorize in terms of scope of data subject to release and time. In this way, agencies cannot assume a right to collect health-related information about such individuals into perpetuity. States are beginning to limit the duration for release authorizations in the absence of set time limits within actual release instruments.

Exhibit 3–3 Example of a HIPAA-Compliant Patient Authorization for Release of Patient Care Records (Spanish language version)

LA CLÍNICA ABC
ANYTOWN, EEUU

AUTORIZACIÓN PARA COMUNICAR INFORMACIÓN MÉDICA PERSONAL (IMP)

Con mi firma abajo, doy permiso para que ABC communique la información médica privada (IMP) de:
Nombre del paciente _____ Fecha del nacimiento _____
Fechas inclusivas de tratamientos _____
Comunique la IMP a: _____ Dirección: _____
Por la razón específica de: _____
Esta autorización incluye la siguiente: __Historia y examen física
__Diagnosis y plan de tratamiento __Medicamentos __Lista de alergias
__Notas progresivas __Sumarios de despedido __Reportajes de rayo-X
__Negativos rayo-X __Resultadas del laboratorio__Reportaje de EKG/EEG
__Papeles de EKG/EEG __Inmunizaciónes __Consultos genéticos
__Otra información (especifíquela): _____
  Comprendo que la IMP comunicada puede incluir información sobre las enfermedades sexuales, el síndrome inmunodeficiente adquirida

(SIDA) o el virus inmunodeficiente humano (VIH), servicios mentales, y el tratamiento para alcoholismo o abuso de drogas.

__Doy permiso para comunicar esta IMP.

__No doy permiso para comunicar esta IMP.

Cualquier uso del IMP del paciente además de el proposito especificado arriba require el permiso del paciente o su representative legal.

Esta autorización es voluntaria. Existe independiente del derecho de tratamiento en ABC. Tengo el derecho de revocar mi autorización en cualquier tiempo. Si revoco esta autorización, tengo que hacerlo en escrito firmado. Tal revocación no se aplica a la IMP ya comuncada según esta autorización. Si no sea revocada, esta autorización se expira en la fecha siguiente, evento o condición: _____. Si no pongo ninguna fecha, evento o condición, esta autorizacion se expira en 90 días después de firmarla.

Tengo el derecho de inspectar o copiar la IMP usada o comunicada, según el CFR 164.524. Comprendo que cualquiera comunicación de información tiene la posibilidad de re-comunicación no autorizada. Mientras que ABC oblige a sus asociados de negocio de cumplir con HIPAA, ABC no puede garantizar su conducta.

Favor de dirigir preguntas sobre la comunicación de la IMP al oficial de la privacidad de la clínica, _____. Gracias.

Firma del paciente o su representativo legal (Diga la relación)   Fecha

Firma del Testigo

Focus on Ethics

R is a social worker at ABC Hospital. Patient S, a 14-year-old minor, reveals to R that S is gay. S elicits and receives R's promise to keep this aspect of S's social history confidential. Nothing about S being gay is documented in S's medical record. Later that day, however, R casually reveals S's confidence to coworkers T, U, and V, during a happy hour social event. Which bases for respecting confidences were violated in this scenario?

CHAPTER SUMMARY

Besides their primary function of creating a ready database of clinically pertinent patient health information, patient care records have important administrative and legal uses, too. They are routinely offered by parties in civil and criminal court cases as substantive evidence of a patient's health status or of the type and quality of care that a patient received. Patient care records are used in virtually every type of administrative and civil legal case, including disability claims cases, workers' compensation cases, personal injury cases, child custody and paternity cases, and healthcare malpractice cases, just to name a few.

Clinical healthcare professionals should always document in patient care records as if the entry were being prepared for court, because such records may in fact find their way into court. A "patient welfare" approach to patient care documentation is recommended over a defensive, self-preservation approach. However, the effective self-protective practice of liability risk management is not necessarily the equivalent of defensive documentation.

Spoliation of records involves the intentional alteration or destruction of patient care entries or records, and there is evidence that this practice is growing among healthcare providers. Documents examiners can easily detect spoliation through gross examination and, where necessary, scientific testing of documents or computer files and systems. If a court finds that a healthcare provider or other healthcare organization employee altered or destroyed records, it will probably order the jury to infer or presume negligence against the provider in a healthcare malpractice case. Punitive damages, not indemnifiable by insurers, may also be awarded against a healthcare provider/organization-defendant in such cases.

A healthcare professional's duty to safeguard confidential patient information is similar to, but not congruous with, the limited healthcare professional–patient privilege against involuntary disclosure of patient information in legal proceedings. All providers and health-related support personnel owe their patients a special duty of confidentiality. It is primarily because of the trust patients have that their healthcare providers will safeguard their confidences that patients are willing to "open up" to providers during examination and intervention. The scope of this ethical and legal duty is governed by state and federal statutory, regulatory, and case law, state licensure and ethical codes, professional association and accreditation standards, and longstanding custom.

The privilege to withhold confidential patient care information in legal proceedings derives from an evidentiary rule that allows a provider covered by federal or state law to refuse to divulge patient examination, evaluative, diagnostic, prognostic, and intervention-related information on behalf of a patient. The privilege being invoked in such cases belongs exclusively to the patient and not to the healthcare provider. Exceptions to confidentiality and privilege may include information pertaining to criminal activity; child, spouse, and elder abuse; and findings related to reportable communicable disease.

NOTES AND REFERENCES

1. Mello M, Chandra A, Gawande A, Studdart D. National costs of the medical liability system. *Health Affairs.* 2010; 29:1569–1577.

2. Hardy CT. Hotline answers. *Physician's Management.* 1992; May:210.

3. In legal terms, an *inference* allows (but does not compel) a conclusion of negligence by a jury based on permissive deductive reasoning that the loss of the patient–plaintiff's treatment records logically occurred at the hands of the defendants, who were at fault. An instruction by a judge to a jury that they are to presume negligence (i.e., a *presumption*) based on lost or altered treatment of records could require the jury to assume negligence unless and until the defendants rebutted the presumption with sufficient evidence of their own to the contrary.

4. See e.g., *Proske v. St. Barnabas Medical Center,* 1998 WL 35297 (N.J. Superior Court Appellate Division, June 23, 1998).

5. Health Care Quality Improvement Act of 1986, 42 United States Code Sections 11101–11152.

6. Prosser RL. Alteration of medical records submitted for legal review. *JAMA.* 1992; 267:2630–2631.

7. Addison L. Establishing the foundation for a spoliation instruction. *Texas Bar Journal.* 2004; June:468–469.

8. *Trevino v. Ortega.* 969 S.W. 2d 950, 952 (Texas 1998).

9. Chase M. How to gain access to your medical files amid varied laws. *Wall Street Journal.* 1996; December 2:B1.

10. Health Insurance Portability and Accountability Act of 1996, Public Law 104191; 45 CFR Parts 160 and 164.

11. 22 TAC Section 165.1b (2010).

12. See 45 CFR 160.103(1)(b). A *business associate* means, with respect to a covered entity, a person who, on behalf of such covered entity, provides legal services involving the disclosure of individually identifiable health information. Accessed July 1, 2010, from www.hipaasurvivalguide.com/hipaa-regulations/160-103.php.

13. A custodian of patient records also has legal recourse if the request for records contained in the *subpoena duces tecum* is overbroad. For example, a request for "all of the patient's medical, dental, and other health records, including billing, payment, and insurance documents for all times, past and current" would be oppressive. The records custodian (medical records administrator) should, through legal counsel, ask the court for a protective order that would require a more tailored subpoena that requests only those records pertinent to conditions related to injuries claimed in the lawsuit. For elucidation on the rights of the records custodian, see Krell BE, Hendrix PL. Protecting the record. *California Lawyer.* 1989; May:86–87.

14. *In Re Doe Grand Jury Proceedings.* No. 97-283-M.P. (Rhode Island Aug. 4, 1998).

15. Federal Rule of Evidence, Section 803(6)(2009), reads: "The following are not excluded by the hearsay rule ... a memorandum, report, record, or data compilation, in any form, of acts, events, conditions, opinions, or diagnoses, made at or near the time by, or from information transmitted by, a person with knowledge, if kept in the course of a regularly conducted business activity, and if it were the regular practice of that business activity to make the memorandum, report, record, or data compilation, all as shown by the testimony of the custodian or other qualified witness, unless the source of information or the method or circumstances of preparation indicate lack of trustworthiness. The term 'business'

as used in this paragraph includes business, institution, association, profession, occupation, and calling of every kind, whether or not conducted for profit."

16. Bok S. *Lying: Moral Choice in Public and Private Life.* New York: Vintage Books; 1989.

17. *Griswold v. Connecticut.* 381 U.S. 479 (1965).

18. *Roe v. Wade.* 410 U.S. 113 (1973).

19. The lead legal case involving a healthcare professional's (psychotherapist) duty to warn third parties of the potential danger of serious bodily harm at the hands of patients under his or her care is *Tarasoff v. Regents of the University of California,* 17 Cal.3d 425, 131 Cal. Rptr. 14,551 P.2d 334 (1976).

20. Indian Health Service, Health Insurance Portability and Accountability Act. Accessed June 16, 2011, from http://www.hipaa.ihs.gov

ADDITIONAL SUGGESTED READINGS

Bergmark RE, Parker M. How confidential is confidential? *Managed Care and Aging.* 1998; 5(1):1–2, 8.

Brous E. Documentation and litigation. *RN.* 2009; 72(2):40–43.

Cohen M. Provera or prozac? Problem handwriting. *Nursing.* 2009; 39(11):15.

Fontenot S. *I Need Some Privacy, Please! Physician-Patient Communication in the Age of HIPAA.* Austin, TX: Texas Medical Association; 2003.

Hall S. *Forensic Text Analysis.* Accessed June 16, 2011, from http://www.ehow.com/facts_6026086_forensic-text-analysis.html

Herman R, Herman S. Understanding spoliation of evidence. *Trial.* 2001; March:45.

Institutional Review Boards and the HIPAA Privacy Rule. *HIPAA Privacy Rule Information for Researchers.* 2003; Aug 15. Accessed June 16, 2011, from http://privacyruleandresearch.nih.gov/pr_02.asp

Knowlton SP. The medical record: Treatment tool or litigation device? *Advances in Skin & Wound Care.* 2003; 16(2):97–98.

Langel S. Averting medical malpractice lawsuits: Effective medicine—or inadequate cure? *Health Affairs.* 2010; 29:1565–1568.

Mandziara v. Canulli. No. 1-97-4644 (Illinois Appellate Court, Sept. 24, 1998) (lawsuit for alleged unauthorized possession of patient mental health records).

Martin R. Falsification of medical records. *Advance for Nurses.* Greater Philadelphia, PA. 2001; June 4:44.

Prost MA. Protecting patient confidentiality. *Advance for Physical Therapists.* 1998; Mar 30:8–10.

Ranke BE. Documentation in the age of litigation. *OT Practice.* 1998; March: 20–24.

Shiffman MA. Law and medicine: Changes in medical records. *International Journal of Cosmetic Surgery and Aesthetic Dermatology.* 2001; 3(3):221–223.

Silber ME, Rabler ME. Access to medical records. *Health Lawyer.* 1996; 8(6): 10–13.

Texas Medical Association. Search term: retention of medical records. Accessed October 4, 2010, from http://www.texmed.org/searchContent.aspx?searchtext=retention%20of%20medical%20records&folderid=1336&searchfor=all&orderby=id&orderdirection=ascending

REVIEW CASE STUDIES

1. You are a registered nurse in charge of the afternoon shift in a surgical intensive care unit. X, a comatose patient in the unit, who is on a respirator, was just arrested and is being transported to the operating room for heart surgery. One of your staff nurses, F, telephones to check on some missing keys, and during the conversation you inform him of patient X's condition. Nurse F suddenly remembers that he forgot to document, in the computerized nursing progress notes during his shift, that he performed respiratory hygiene and postural drainage on patient X twice during his shift. He asks you to add that information to his end-of-shift note. What do you tell him?

2. J, a paralegal employed by WXY Law Associates, telephones your office requesting the name, address, and other personal and clinical information about a patient being treated in your clinic for soft tissue injuries sustained in a motor vehicle accident. J claims that he has been in contact with the patient about pursuing a product liability class action lawsuit stemming from a defective automobile part. You are personally familiar with the named patient J seeks information about. Should you release any information to the paralegal?

3. You are the medical librarian at AZ Community Hospital. While conducting a research computer search, you overhear two teenage summer volunteers from the community health office talking to one another about the HIV status of a patient in the facility. You

do not hear the patient's name and are not sure that any name was used. What course of action should you take?

DISCUSSION: REVIEW CASE STUDIES

1. You should inform nurse F that you cannot add information to his prior treatment documentation. Whether electronically or handwritten, intentional alteration of prior documentation entries constitutes illegal spoliation of records. Spoliation can usually be detected by document examiners, even when performed on a computer. If you agree with nurse F to alter his documentation of patient X's care, then you may be liable for "conspiracy" as well as spoliation. If it is critical for nurse F to add the information about patient X's respiratory care performed earlier that day, then nurse F should personally document his prior omission as a new entry. Before doing so in this case, however, nurse F may want to coordinate with the hospital risk manager, because patient X's condition has deteriorated and patient X's case may become a lawsuit.

2. You should refrain from providing any information to J under the circumstances of this hypothetical case for several reasons. First, although J's employer may have formed an attorney–client relationship with the patient in issue, you are not a party to that agreement. You have a separate legal duty to safeguard the patient's personal information from unlawful disclosure to others. Although some state statutes may allow for unilateral release of nonclinical information about patients to third parties, it would probably be imprudent to do so in today's litigious environment. In addition, HIPAA disallows such disclosure without the patient's signed written authorization. Even if the patient had given proper HIPAA authorization for release of PHI, J's request for information was made over the telephone. *Never give patient information out to anyone over the telephone.* J's request must be made in writing and should appear on his attorney's letterhead to reference the source of the request. Release only that information within the scope of the patient's authorization and not necessarily all that has been asked for by J.

3. The volunteers have disclosed, in public, private facts about a patient. As librarian, you probably have no official need or right to know such information. This invasion of privacy probably will not be legally actionable, however, if the patient cannot be identified, or if others, besides the librarian—a hospital employee—did not overhear the volunteers' conversation. If the patient can somehow be identified (by the volunteers' description of the patient, for example), and if the patient sues and wins, then the hospital probably will be vicariously liable for damages suffered by the patient for the volunteers' invasion of privacy.

For the Suggested Answer Framework to the Focus on Ethics, please refer to Appendix D.

CHAPTER 4

Patient Care Record Informed Consent Documentation Issues

This chapter examines the concept of patient informed consent, as it relates to healthcare examination and intervention. The history of the development of the law of informed consent is presented, along with the sources of authority for requiring patient informed consent in healthcare settings. A standardized checklist of disclosure elements for ethical and legally sufficient informed consent is offered, with the caveat that this information is illustrative and not necessarily a reflection of the law of any particular state. The chapter ends with a discussion of documentation guidelines for memorializing patient informed consent.

INTRODUCTION

The issue of patient informed consent to examination and intervention is one that is or should be of critical concern to all healthcare professionals, whether they examine and intervene on behalf of patients with or without a referral from another provider. There are relatively few healthcare malpractice cases solely involving allegations of lack of informed consent. However, with current practice trends and issues, including direct access to patients for nonphysician primary healthcare professionals from many disciplines, the time constraints of managed healthcare delivery, and the renewed focus on core values and ethical responsibilities, the issue of informed consent is made all the more salient.

All primary healthcare providers have an ethical and a legal duty to provide their patients with sufficient disclosure information about examination and interventions to allow them to make a knowing, intelligent, and unequivocal decision regarding whether or not to accept patient care offered to them. The concept of informed consent is premised on respect for the patient's rights of autonomy and self-determination (i.e., the inherent right of every patient with legal and mental capacity [or of a legitimate surrogate decision-maker] to control the healthcare decision-making process and decide the intervention(s), if any, that will be carried out on him or her).

LEGAL RECOGNITION OF THE CONCEPT OF INFORMED CONSENT

Informed consent to healthcare intervention is recognized as a fundamental right in case law,[1] by statute, or as a matter of customary practice in virtually every jurisdiction. It is also recognized as such a right by health professional practice, ethics, and healthcare organization/system accreditation standards.

A number of state legislatures have enacted statutory informed consent procedures that include informed consent forms, signed by patients, for specific surgeries and other medical procedures. A patient's signature on such a form may constitute presumptive legal evidence of patient informed consent. When such a statute is in effect in an informed consent–based healthcare malpractice case, the patient must usually prove that consent was induced by a misrepresentation of material facts or must produce credible evidence that he or she did not reasonably understand the form in order to rebut such a presumption.

U.S. Supreme Court case decisions interpreting the Constitution also reflect respect for patient self-determination in making important healthcare decisions. Case law based on the federal constitutional right of privacy has balanced patient autonomy against "compelling state interests" and frequently has ruled in favor of patients and/or their surrogate decision-makers on issues such as the withdrawal of life and nutritional support.

Health professional associations have promulgated rules and standards concerning patient informed consent. The Focus on Ethics exercise later in this chapter offers readers an opportunity to explore, compare, and contrast several primary disciplines' informed consent ethical provisions.

The federal Patient Self-Determination Act of 1990 also codifies the rights of patients to control healthcare decision-making, both routine and extraordinary. The law binds hospitals, long-term care facilities, and other healthcare facilities participating in Medicare and Medicaid to its provisions.

The Patient Self-Determination Act provides in pertinent part[2] that

The requirement of this subsection is that a provider . . . maintain written policies and procedures with respect to all adult individuals receiving medical care. . .

To provide written information to each such individual concerning an individual's rights under State law (whether statutory or as recognized by the courts of the state) to make decisions concerning . . . medical care, including the right to accept or refuse medical or surgical treatment.

Some authorities argue that financial reimbursement for healthcare services should be tied to proof that the patient (or surrogate decision-maker) gave valid informed consent to treatment.

EVOLUTION OF THE LAW OF INFORMED CONSENT

The concept of patient informed consent is largely a result of the consumer rights movement that has swept the Western world since World War II, although it was recognized earlier. In 1914, a respected jurist, Justice Benjamin Cardozo, wrote in his opinion in the case of *Schloendorff v. Society of New York Hospital* that "every human being of adult years and sound mind has a right to determine what shall be done with his own body; and a surgeon who performs an operation without his patient's consent commits an assault for which he is liable in damages."[3]

For several decades after the Schloendorff decision, the care of patients without their consent was treated as an assault or battery, depending on the term used by the particular state. By definition, an *assault* normally encompasses intentional conduct on the part of one person that creates in another an apprehension or anticipation of the application of force. In other words, an assault is a fear of an unwanted touch. The actual application of force, in the form of an unconsented, unprivileged harmful or offensive touch or other physical contact is, in legal terms, a *battery*. Commonly recognized examples of commission of a battery in the healthcare setting include striking a patient in anger, amputating the wrong limb, excising the wrong breast in a mastectomy during surgery, or administering an ultrasound treatment in the wrong situs.

> **Assault:** the apprehension or anticipation of the application of unauthorized physical force.
> **Battery:** the unconsented, unprivileged harmful or offensive touching of another person.
> **Sexual assault or battery:** the unconsented, unprivileged, harmful, or offensive intentional touching, or attempted touching, of the sexual or other intimate parts of another person, for the purpose of sexual arousal or gratification (of either party), or for patient abuse.

For many years, allegations of a lack of patient informed consent continued to be treated as the intentional torts of assault and battery. The precise term *informed consent* only came into common use after it was used by the Kansas Supreme Court in the case of *Natanson v. Kline.* That case concerned a claim by a cancer patient that she was injured by excessive radiation therapy. The patient claimed that she did not understand the nature and consequences of the treatment, and if she had, she would not have consented to it. The justice writing the legal opinion in *Natanson* stated:[4]

> The fundamental distinction between assault and battery on one hand, and negligence such as would constitute malpractice, on the other, is that the former is intentional and the latter unintentional. . . .

> We are here concerned with a case where the patient consented to the treatment, but alleges in a malpractice action that the nature and consequences of the risks of the treatment were not properly explained to her. This relates directly to whether the physician has obtained the *informed consent* [emphasis added] of the patient to render the treatment administered. . . .

> The courts frequently state that the relation(ship) between the physician and his patient is a fiduciary one, and therefore the physician has an obligation to make a full and frank disclosure to the patient of all pertinent facts related to his illness. We are here concerned with a case where the physician is charged with treating the patient without consent on the ground the patient was not fully informed of the nature of the treatment or its consequences, and, therefore, any "consent" obtained was ineffective. . . .

In considering the obligation of a physician to disclose and explain to the patient, in language as simple as necessary, the nature of the ailment, the nature of the proposed treatment, the probability of success or of alternatives, and, perhaps, the risks of unfortunate results and unforeseen conditions within the body, we do not think the administration of such an obligation, by imposing liability for malpractice if the treatment were administered without such explanation, where explanation would reasonably be made, presents any insurmountable obstacles.

The appellate court in *Natanson* reversed the trial level court's jury verdict in favor of the defendants and ordered a retrial with instructions to be given by the trial judge about a physician's duty to make disclosures about a patient's illness; the nature of the recommended intervention; and its risks, expected benefits, and alternative interventions to ensure patient informed consent. *Natanson* was one of the first cases to properly label the treatment of a patient without informed consent as health professional negligence, instead of calling it a battery.

In another landmark informed consent case, *Canterbury v. Spence*, the federal appeals court refined the concept of informed consent even more and established a new standard for information disclosure by healthcare providers to patients. In *Canterbury*, which involved a laminectomy patient's claim that the surgeon negligently failed to inform him fully of postoperative complications, Judge Spotswood Robinson III held[5] that:

The patient's reliance upon the physician is a trust of the kind which traditionally has exacted obligations beyond those associated with arms length transactions. [The patient's] dependence upon the physician for information affecting his well-being, in terms of contemplated treatment, is well-nigh abject. . . .

We now find, as a part of the physician's overall obligation to the patient, a similar duty of reasonable disclosure of the choices with respect to proposed therapy and the dangers inherently and potentially involved. . . .

The topics importantly demanding a communication of information are the inherent and potential hazards of the proposed treatment, the alternatives to that treatment, if any, and the results likely if the patient remains untreated. The factors contributing significance to the dangerousness of a medical treatment are, of course, the incidence of injury and the degree of harm threatened. A very small chance of death or serious disablement may well be significant; a potential disability which dramatically outweighs the potential benefit of the therapy or the detriments of the existing malady may summon discussion with the patient.

There is no bright line separating the significant from the insignificant; the answer in any case must abide a rule of reason.

Judge Robinson reversed a trial court *directed* [expedited] *verdict* for the defendants (surgeon and hospital) and ordered a new trial. The *Canterbury* case is revisited in later sections, during discussion of prerequisites to legal action for an allegation of a lack of informed consent, exceptions to the requirement to obtain a patient's informed consent before examination or intervention, and the legal and professional ethical standards for information disclosure.

The *Natanson* and *Canterbury* cases, then, established that the failure on the part of a healthcare provider to obtain a patient's informed consent to examination or intervention is health professional negligence and not the intentional tort of assault or battery. Care of a patient without the patient's informed consent means that the patient was not given sufficient disclosure information about the process by his or her primary healthcare provider to make an intelligent, informed choice about whether or not to agree to it.

> Failure on the part of a healthcare provider to obtain a patient's informed consent before examination or intervention is a form of health professional negligence, and constitutes substandard care delivery.

WHEN IS THE FAILURE TO OBTAIN PATIENT INFORMED CONSENT LEGALLY ACTIONABLE?

Although every failure to obtain patient informed consent before examination or intervention is professional negligence (absent some recognized exception to the requirement), not every such breach of duty can result in legal action by the patient. Litigation over informed consent only arises when the following occur:

1. An undisclosed risk materializes, resulting in injury to the patient.

2. The patient establishes (i.e., proves) that he or she would not have consented to examination or intervention had the risk been disclosed.

The court in *Canterbury* discussed the requirement for a causal connection between patient injury and the negligent failure to impart information to the patient, and reasoned the following:

> No more than breach of any other legal duty does nonfulfillment of the physician's obligation to disclose alone establish liability to the patient. *An unrevealed risk that should have been made known must materialize, for otherwise the omission, however unpardonable, is legally without consequence. Occurrence of the risk must be harmful to the patient, for negligence unrelated to injury is nonactionable* [emphasis added]. And, as in malpractice actions generally, there must be a causal relationship between the physician's failure to adequately divulge and damage to the patient.
>
> *A causal connection exists when, but only when, disclosure of significant risks incidental to treatment would have resulted in a decision against it* [emphasis added]. The patient obviously has no complaint if he would have submitted to the therapy notwithstanding awareness that the risk was one of its perils. On the other hand, the very purpose of the disclosure rule is to protect the patient against the consequences which, if known, he would have avoided by forgoing the treatment.

Litigation concerning informed consent should never have to occur, because obtaining a patient's informed consent is an ethical and legal prerequisite to examination and intervention. And because the elemental requirements for gaining a patient's informed consent are relatively straightforward, the process is not particularly burdensome for clinicians. Providers simply need to make informed consent an integral part of their patient examinations and intervention processes.

DISCLOSURE ELEMENTS FOR LEGALLY SUFFICIENT PATIENT INFORMED CONSENT

The following elements normally must be disclosed to the patient before examination or intervention, then patient (or surrogate) questions must be actively solicited by, and any questions that the patient has, satisfactorily answered by a primary healthcare provider to meet the legal requirements for patient informed consent. The exact requirements for informed consent vary from state to state. The list that follows does not necessarily represent the law of any particular state. (See your facility or personal attorney for specific advice.)

Patient informed consent to examination involves disclosure and discussion of the patient's medical or other prior relevant diagnosis and the parameters of the intended examination. For a patient's consent to substantive intervention to be legally sufficient, or "informed," the primary healthcare provider must relate the following elements to the patient in layperson's language at the level of patient understanding:

1. A description of the patient's health problem (diagnosis or evaluative findings) and the recommended intervention(s).

2. Material risks, if any, associated with the recommended intervention. Material risks include important "decisional" risks (including foreseeable complications associated with the recommended intervention that are, or should be important to the patient) or precautions that would cause an ordinary, reasonable patient to think carefully when deciding whether to undergo or reject the recommended intervention.

3. Reasonable alternatives, if any, to the proposed intervention(s) (i.e., other effective potential interventions that would be acceptable substitutes under legal standards of practice). The provider must be sure to include discussion of the relative risks and benefits of alternative interventions.

4. Expected benefits, or goals, and prognosis associated with the recommended intervention(s).

Providers should memorize the above elements and routinely cover each of them with every patient. After the applicable disclosure elements are imparted to a patient, the healthcare provider must solicit patient questions and answer them to the patient's satisfaction before proceeding on to either examination or intervention.

When the English language is not a patient's primary language (or that of the surrogate decision-maker, for patients lacking mental or physical capacity), the provider must use the services of an interpreter to ensure patient comprehension of the informed consent disclosure elements. Careful documentation is recommended whenever an interpreter is employed during these processes. An example of documenting the services of an interpreter during informed consent disclosure appears in **Exhibit 4–1**.

Exhibit 4–1 Example of Informed Consent Documentation Involving an Interpreter for the Patient

ABC General Hospital
Rehabilitation Center, Physical Therapy Section
May 23, 201x /1600

S: 42 y o F, dx multiple sclerosis, wheelchair-bound, referred for "evaluation, facilitative range of motion, and progressive exercise and ambulation, to tolerance." Pt. is Spanish-speaking; Mrs. Gonzales, Red Cross volunteer, acted as interpreter.

0: . . .

A: . . .

P: Begin AAROM today; standing at parallel bars, to tolerance. I obtained informed consent from the pt. in Spanish through Mrs. Gonzales, interpreter.   Pt. verbalizes understanding of her diagnosis and my examination findings; the recommended intervention as outlined in Dr. Doe's order; the risks of muscle soreness, fatigue, and the slight risk of joint subluxation associated with exercise; and information about the alternative options of bed rest and limited activity in her wheelchair. I asked for her questions, through Mrs. Gonzales. She wanted to know how long sessions lasted; I told her 45 min to 1 hr. each, but only to her tolerance. She verbalized satisfaction with the program as outlined and agreed to try it.

G: . . .

—**Reggie Hausenfus, PT, #07165733**

Checklist Disclosure Elements for Patient Informed Consent to Intervention

- Evaluative findings and/or diagnosis (or diagnoses)
- Description of the recommended intervention(s)
- Material (decisional) risks of possible harm or foreseeable complications associated with the recommended intervention(s)
- Expected benefits (goals) and prognosis
- Reasonable alternatives to the recommended intervention(s), including relative risks, benefits, and prognosis associated with these reasonable alternative interventions
- Solicit and answer the patient questions, in a language, and at a level of comprehension that the patient understands.

As primary healthcare providers, always bear in mind that <u>any</u> health-related intervention is only a recommended intervention (even if prescribed or ordered by another healthcare professional), unless and until a patient having mental and legal capacity (directly, or through a surrogate decision-maker) agrees to it.

DOCUMENTING A PATIENT'S "INFORMED REFUSAL" OF AN INTERVENTION

In the event that a patient is inclined to refuse examination and/or intervention altogether, the primary healthcare professional involved in the patient's care must undertake a further step to meet legal requirements for informed consent. In cases involving patient declination of care, a provider must explain to the patient, in an objective fashion, the expected consequences of refusing examination and/or intervention. After such disclosure, a decision by the patient to refuse care would constitute legally *informed refusal*. Careful and thorough documentation in the patient care record of the previous processes, in informed refusal situations, is always required in case a legal action ensues. An example of how to document patient informed refusal of intervention appears in **Exhibit 4–2**.

Exhibit 4–2 Example of Documentation of Patient Informed Refusal of Intervention

ABC General Hospital
Rehabilitation Center, Physical Therapy Section
May 23, 201x/1600

S: 42 v o F, dx multiple sclerosis, wheelchair-bound, referred for "evaluation, facilitative range of motion, and progressive exercise and ambulation, to tolerance."

O: ...

A: ...

P: Begin AAROM today; standing at parallel bars, to tolerance. After explanation to pt. of her diagnosis and my evaluative findings; the proposed therapy as outlined in Dr. Doe's order; the risks of muscle soreness, fatigue, and the slight risk of joint subluxation associated with exercise; and the alternative options of bed rest and limited activity in her wheelchair, pt. stated, "I don't want any treatment." I explained to her, in the presence of Holly Wood, PT, the risks of joint contractures, muscle wasting, osteoporosis, and cardiovascular compromise associated with inactivity, and invited her questions about the recommended intervention and my explanation of the risks of forgoing intervention. She still refused to proceed. Pt. transported back to nursing floor; RN in charge and Dr. Doe notified. Will attempt to persuade pt. to change her mind in the A.M.

—Reggie Hausenfus, PT, #07165733

Checklist Disclosure Elements for Patient Informed Refusal of Intervention

- Examination and evaluative findings, diagnosis.
- Description of the recommended intervention.

- Material (decisional) risks of possible harm associated with the recommended intervention.
- Expected benefits and prognosis.
- Reasonable alternatives, and their relative benefits and risks.
- Solicit and satisfactorily answer patient questions.
- Explain the foreseeable consequences of refusing intervention.
- Carefully and thoroughly document the foregoing processes in the patient care record.
- Communicate expeditiously with the referring entity, if any.

CLINICAL MODELS FOR IMPLEMENTING INFORMED CONSENT

Healthcare professionals may feel a sense of frustration with having the responsibility of going through a litany of checklist elements to obtain patient informed consent for each one of their patients, especially in the hurried world of managed (or as some might say, minimal) care. Providers may also be confused about how to document in patient care records the fact that patient informed consent has been obtained. Rozovsky[6] correctly asserts that informed consent is a *process* and not just the *pro forma* adherence to oral or written checklists or preprinted forms. Checklists and careful documentation about patient informed consent, although important, only serve as some evidence that this critically important process took place. That process is ensuring, through good communication, that a patient truly understands the parameters of a proposed treatment and agrees to accept examination and/or intervention.

Documentation of patient informed consent, although important, is only partial evidence that the critical process of communication between healthcare provider and patient took place, and that the patient truly understood the parameters of examination and/or recommended intervention and agreed to it.

Several recognized models can be adopted by healthcare providers to implement patient informed consent. The rules-oriented legalistic model and the traditional medical model focus on strict compliance with regulatory or health professional practice standards, and not on patient autonomy over healthcare decision-making. The normative model focuses on the patient's right to self-determination so much that it defers to patient choice in all circumstances, even when that choice is seemingly irrational. The interactive model, advocated in various forms by the author, and by Katz,[7] Rozovsky,[6] and others, is the patient informed consent model that focuses attention on the following processes of:

- Communication between provider and patient
- Patient comprehension and education
- Patient participation in, and joint responsibility for, healthcare decision-making

This model, grounded in mutual trust and respect, recognizes that healthcare providers and patients come together both as equals and non-equals. Although providers normally come into the process with a greater understanding of scientific principles concerning health and disease, their patients usually possess a greater intuition about their own personal health status. Therefore, this model offers the best opportunity, through shared decision-making, to simultaneously improve the quality of patient care delivery and manage the formidable risk of healthcare malpractice exposure incident to clinical practice.

SPECIAL INFORMED CONSENT ISSUES

Who Must Obtain a Patient's Informed Consent?

Any primary healthcare provider who provides care for a patient has a legal and professional ethical duty to obtain the patient's informed consent before commencing examination or intervention. For non-physician primary healthcare providers, this duty applies whether or not the provider cares for patients with a physician (or other provider) referral. Referring physicians often issue generic referral orders such as "evaluate and treat" and, therefore, practically cannot ascertain the precise interventions that a nonphysician consultant will employ. Also, nonphysician primary healthcare provider-specialist consultants typically know more about their practices than do referring entities and are therefore in a better position to explain them to patients and answer patient questions.

> It is primary healthcare professionals who bear legal and professional ethical responsibility for gaining patients' informed consent, not referral entities, nor assistants, aides, clerical personnel, or others. This point is particularly important to remember in the managed care environment, in which many care extenders may participate.

A healthcare organization or system may bear vicarious or primary liability for the failure of providers in its facilities to obtain patient's informed consent to examinations and interventions. In addition to being indirectly liable for the conduct of professional employee staff, healthcare organizations have an independent primary duty to establish practice standards and monitor patient care within their facilities, irrespective of who delivers that care.

How Often Must Informed Consent Be Obtained?

Must informed consent be obtained over and over again for the same patient before each individual intervention? No. Renewed informed consent only needs to be obtained when an original intervention plan is substantially changed or substituted with another plan of care.

Substitute Healthcare Providers and the Need for Renewal of Informed Consent

What are the informed consent responsibilities, if any, of substitute providers who take over for a primary healthcare provider who goes away to a continuing education course or on vacation? In a hospital setting, a patient may not have an expectation of exclusive care by a single non-physician provider in a clinical setting, so that informed consent gained by one provider is valid so long as a substitute provider carries out the same program.

In a private practice setting, however, such as an outpatient physical or occupational therapy clinic, a provider responsible for vacation or other coverage may not be able to rely on the original therapist's disclosure of information and receipt of patient informed consent to intervention, particularly when documentation of informed consent is absent or insufficient to rely on. Under such circumstances, it is advisable to gain patient informed consent independently and document it before providing care for the patient. (This is a gray area in the law of informed consent, without many reported cases.) An example of how to document informed consent as a substitute provider in an outpatient clinical setting appears in **Exhibit 4–3**.

Exhibit 4–3 Example of Documentation of Informed Consent by a Substitute Healthcare Provider

ABC General Hospital
Rehabilitation Center, Physical Therapy Section
May 26, 201x/1600

S: 42 y o F, dx multiple sclerosis, wheelchair-bound, referred on May 23, 201x, for "evaluation, facilitative range of motion, and progressive exercise and ambulation, to tolerance." Has been to PT Clinic for last 2 days and was treated by Reggie Hausenfus, PT, who had to take emergency vacation to attend his father's funeral. Pt. appears confused by my substitute coverage of PT care.

O: . . .

A: . . .

P: Renewed pt. I/C by explaining my examination/evaluative findings; diagnosis; the course of therapy as outlined in Dr. Doe's order and R. Hausenfus' progress notes; the risks of muscle soreness, fatigue, and the slight risk of joint subluxation associated with exercise; and the alternative options of bed rest and limited activity in her wheelchair. I asked for her questions. She had none and stated that she now understood why another therapist was caring for her today. Cont. w/ program, as outlined. Tolerated 45-min session well.

G: . . .

—**Carrie Cover, PT, #07263720**

EXCEPTIONS TO THE REQUIREMENTS FOR INFORMED CONSENT

Are there any exceptions to the legal requirement to obtain a patient's informed consent before treatment? Yes.

One exception to informed consent is the *emergency doctrine*, under which consent is typically not obtained for emergency lifesaving care. This doctrine applies when, for example, a clinical provider performs cardio-pulmonary resuscitation on a patient who suffers a myocardial infarction while in the provider's clinic. Under these circumstances, patient consent generally is presumed. Exceptions to this exception include valid patient advance (or surrogate agent) directives and do-not-resuscitate orders disallowing intervention.

A rare exception to informed consent is *therapeutic privilege*, under which a healthcare provider may be excused from disclosing information to a patient who, in the provider's professional judgment, could not psychologically cope with the information disclosed (e.g., when the diagnosis or prognosis involves a life-threatening disease).

Situations that involves a qualification, but not an exception, to the doctrine of informed consent include the care of minors (who lack *legal capacity*) and of adults lacking mental capacity, and under conservatorship or guardianship because of such a condition. Informed consent in such circumstances is obtained from a legally appointed surrogate decision-maker and not from the patient. An exception to the no-legal-capacity rule for minors involves minors' rights in some states to make independent decisions concerning such conditions as pregnancy and intervention for drug and alcohol addiction and for venereal disease interventions.

STANDARDS FOR DISCLOSURE

There are two basic legal standards for disclosure of information for informed consent. Some states employ the professional standard of disclosure, meaning that a healthcare provider must disclose to the patient that information that another provider of the same profession, acting under the same or similar circumstances, would have disclosed. Legal cases tried in professional-standard jurisdictions often require expert testimony about the information that a defendant's professional peers would consider appropriate for disclosure.

A number of states use a layperson's standard for disclosure. In these states, a provider must disclose all the information that an ordinary, reasonable patient under the same circumstances would deem material in making an informed decision.

The court in *Canterbury* delineated the two standards as follows:

> The larger number of courts, as might be expected, have applied tests framed with reference to prevailing fashion within the medical profession. Some have measured the disclosure by "good medical practice," others what a reasonable practitioner would have bared under the circumstances, and still others by what medical custom in the community would demand. We have explored this rather considerable body of law but are unprepared to follow it. . . .

> In our view, the patient's right of self-decision shapes the boundaries of the duty to reveal. That right can be effectively exercised only if the patient possesses enough information to enable an intelligent choice. The scope of the physician's communication to the patient, then, must be measured by the patient's need and that need is the materiality to the patient's decision: all risks potentially affecting the decision must be unmasked. And to safeguard the patient's interest in achieving his own determination on treatment, the law must itself set the standard for adequate disclosure.

> Optimally for the patient, exposure of a risk would be mandatory whenever the patient would deem it significant to his decision, either singly or in combination with other risks. Such a requirement, however, would summon the physician to second-guess the patient, whose ideas on materiality could hardly be known to the physician. . . . Consonantly with orthodox negligence doctrine, the physician's liability for nondisclosure is to be determined on the basis of foresight, not hindsight; no less than any other aspect of negligence, the issue of nondisclosure must be approached from the viewpoint of the reasonableness of the physician's divulgence in terms of what he knows or should know to be the patient's informational needs. If, but only if, the fact-finder can say that the physician's communication was unreasonably inadequate is an imposition of liability legally or morally justified. . . .

> From these considerations we derive the breadth of the disclosure of risks legally to be required. The scope of the standard is not subjective as to either the physician or the patient; it remains objective with due regard for the patient's informational needs and with suitable leeway for the physician's situation. In broad outline, we agree that "a risk is thus material when a

reasonable person, in what the physician knows or should know to be in the patient's position, would be likely to attach significance to the risk or cluster of risks in deciding whether or not to forego the proposed therapy."

The topics importantly demanding a communication of information are

- The inherent and potential hazards of the proposed treatment
- The alternatives to that treatment, if any
- The results likely if the patient remains untreated

The factors contributing significance to the dangerousness of a medical technique are, of course, the incidence of injury and the degree of the harm threatened. A very small chance of death or serious disablement may well be significant; a potential disability which dramatically outweighs the potential benefit of the therapy or the detriments of the existing malady may [warrant] discussion with the patient.

There is no bright line separating the significant from the insignificant; the answer in any case must abide a rule of reason. Some dangers—infection, for example—are inherent in any operation; there is no obligation to communicate those of which persons of average sophistication are aware. Even more clearly, the physician bears *no responsibility for discussion of hazards the patient has already discovered or those having no apparent materiality to the patient's decision on therapy* [emphasis added].

Canterbury, then, was the first reported case to change the focus of inquiry in an informed consent–based healthcare malpractice case from what a reasonable healthcare provider would disclose to a patient to what an ordinary, reasonable, prudent patient would expect to hear about a recommended intervention: its relative risks, benefits, and effect on prognosis, and similar information about reasonable alternatives, if any.

INFORMED CONSENT IN THE SPECIALTY OR LIMITED PRACTICE SETTING: PREVENTING AN ALLEGATION OF PATIENT ABANDONMENT

The issue of liability for patient abandonment is discussed in greater detail in Chapter 6; however, there are informed consent issues involving providers practicing in a specialty or limited practice setting that warrant mentioning in this section.

Legally actionable abandonment of a patient occurs when a healthcare provider improperly unilaterally terminates a professional relationship with a patient. Providers practicing in specialty areas, such as physicians who confine their practices to cosmetic or other types of surgery, or physical therapists who limit their practices to orthopedic or sports physical therapy, need to carefully apprise their patients of the restricted nature of their practices. Then, when the surgery is completed, or the zenith of the patient's rehabilitation has been reached, the specialist can more easily disengage from further care for unrelated patient complaints.

If a claim or lawsuit ensues, alleging patient abandonment, thorough documentation of the patient's informed consent to limited scope care may be crucial to avoid healthcare malpractice liability. An example of how to document patient informed consent to care in a limited scope specialty practice appears in **Exhibit 4–4**.

Exhibit 4–4 Example of Documentation of Informed Consent by a Healthcare Provider in a Specialty (Limited) Practice Setting

Doe Occupational Health Center Specializing in Evaluation and Treatment of Hand Disorders, Halifax, Nova Scotia, Canada Dec. 1, 201x/1935

S: 32 y o F, ceramics artist, referred by Dr. Smith for "evaluation and gentle, progressive mobilization, left hand, s/p immobilization of left hand X 6 wks. for suspected scaphoid fx. No fx."

O: . . .

A: . . .

P: Paraffin rx X 20 min q.d., F/B gentle mobilization, AROM, and mild PREs, to tolerance. I/C to rx obtained. Pt. advised that mine is a limited scope practice, specializing exclusively in hand therapy. Pt. asked if I could evaluate her R shoulder also, which cracks w/ shoulder AROM X 3 yrs. Pt. is 3 yrs. s/p L CVA. I told her that a separate referral would be required for an OT or PT to evaluate her R shoulder and that I did not work with patients with shoulder complaints because of the limited scope of my practice to hand care. She verbalized understanding and agreed to seek a referral from Dr. Smith for OT or PT evaluation of her R shoulder at ABC Hospital.

G: . . .

—Aidee El, OT

INFORMED CONSENT AS A RISK MANAGEMENT TOOL FOR PREVENTING ALLEGATIONS OF BATTERY AND SEXUAL BATTERY

Unlike most other professional–client relationships, the delivery of health care routinely involves "hands-on" therapy or other intervention. In some disciplines—medicine and surgery, physical, occupational and speech therapy, nursing, and chiropractic, among others—these manual procedures can be very intensive and occasionally uncomfortable. With techniques such as deep friction massage, myofascial mobilization, and spinal, pelvic, and extremity manipulation, clinicians may work close to patients' private zones (i.e., breasts, buttocks, and genitalia). It is imperative that a patient fully understand any manual therapy procedure before undergoing therapy and give his or her informed consent to it.

Of the growing number of sexual battery allegations lodged by patients against primary healthcare providers, many, perhaps, are simply the result of a lack of understanding or a misunderstanding about the nature of the procedure used on the patient. A caring, prudent provider must take the time to explain manual therapy procedures carefully and thoroughly to a patient for whom they are prescribed; solicit and answer any patient questions; and address any patient concerns before, during, or after these procedures. It is especially important to let patients know they have the absolute right to order a halt to any intervention (from massage, to joint mobilization, to functional or work capacity evaluation) at any time, for any reason. It is critically important, anytime intensive hands-on manual therapy is to be carried out in the vicinity of a patient's private zones of contact, to thoroughly document the informed consent elements explained to the patient in the patient care record. An example of documentation of informed consent for physical therapy manipulation appears in **Exhibit 4–5.**

Exhibit 4–5 Example of Documentation of Informed Consent for Intensive Hands-On Physical Therapy Intervention (to Prevent a Sexual Battery Allegation)

M&M Community Hospital, Physical Therapy Center
Aug. 5, 201x/1315

S: 32 y o F, referred by Dr. Ella for "evaluation and consideration for myofascial mobilization for R sternoclavicular pain X 2 months; s/p sling immobilization X 4 wks for recurrent ant. sh. dislocation." Med. hx includes 3 X recurrent ant. shoulder dislocations secondary to FOOSH; psychiatric treatment last Dec. for depression. No prior surgeries. Meds include Elavil, Norflex, and Motrin.

O: Point tenderness over R S-C joint and over medial R chest. FAROM. . . .

A: R sternoclavicular myofascial pain syndrome, secondary to sling immobilization. R breast pathology ruled out by Dr. Ella, per telephonic discussion of pt.'s exam.

P: R sternoclavicular manual myofascial mobilization, including transverse friction massage and joint mobilization. Reviewed informed consent elements with patient and her husband, as follows: (1) explanation of dx, R sternoclavicular myofascial pain syndrome, secondary to sling immobilization; (2) proposed rx, R sternoclavicular manual myofascial mobilization, transverse friction massage, and R S-C joint mobilization. Demonstrated technique on myself for pt. and husband; (3) material risks: possible soft tissue tenderness and bruising and discomfort with chest & BUE AROM; and (4) reasonable alternatives/adjuncts to mobilization: heat, cryotherapy, and stretching ROM. Pt. had question about intensity of pain during rx. I told her she should only experience mild discomfort and should tell me if she experiences any more degree of discomfort, and I will modify my pressure. She and husband understand all; pt. consents to Rx as proposed. Conducted 15-min myofascial mobilization session w/ pt. Mrs. Jones, Red Cross volunteer, present during initial session. Pt. had no adverse reaction to initial intervention.

G: . . .

—**Tom Fields, PT, OCS**

INFORMED CONSENT DOCUMENTATION FORMATS

Like other issues in the law of informed consent, the legally correct form for documenting a patient's informed consent to examination and intervention varies from state to state. Some states have specific statutory disclosure requirements for medical and/or surgical procedures and may consider statutory form disclosure presumptive—or even conclusive (irrefutable)— evidence of a patient's informed consent. Other states permit the use of a wide variety of methods for documenting informed consent. (This discussion is intended to be informational and not dispositive on the law of any particular state. Ask your legal counsel whether the form of documentation you use in your clinical practice is legally acceptable in your state, and if it is appropriate for your practice setting and circumstances.)

There are many acceptable ways to document patients' informed consent. As a premise, it should be said that primary healthcare professionals must always use some means of memorializing, through documentation, that their patients give their informed consent before examination and intervention. This section illustrates several commonly used methods of documenting patient informed consent to intervention, including use of "boilerplate" consent forms, documentation in shorthand and longhand form in patient care records, use of informed consent checklists, and reference to standard operating procedures or broad clinic policy statements.

Boilerplate (Standardized) Consent Forms

There are two types of consent forms: short and long. Both forms are signed (and often each element is initialed) by the patient. The short form simply lists the required components of informed consent, followed by the patient's, provider's, and witness' signatures. Such a format might read as follows:

> I, John Patient, was informed of my examination/evaluative findings, diagnosis, prognosis, and recommended intervention(s) and material risks of possible harm. My questions were solicited and answered to my satisfaction. I give my informed consent to the recommended interventions of my primary healthcare provider.
>
> Patient Signature
>
> Provider Signature
>
> Witness Signature

A long consent form may be customized for individual patients and may include specifics about each element of required disclosure. Because the provider is legally bound by whatever appears—or does not appear— on the long consent form, the legal danger of the use of such a form is that an element of disclosure, especially including procedure-related material risks, might be inadvertently omitted from the form. The fact that the provider might, in fact, have imparted the missing information verbally to the patient might not withstand legal scrutiny in an informed consent–based healthcare malpractice action. An additional consideration in using the long form is the fact that it is relatively time-consuming to complete, making its use under managed care especially unattractive and impractical.

There are recognized problems with standardized patient consent forms (i.e., hospital admission blanket consent forms), some of which can render them legally ineffective as evidence of patient informed consent to treatment. Often, these forms are overly broad or ambiguous. Often drafted by attorneys or administrators, many of these forms cannot be understood by lay people, that is, by patients. In such cases, courts almost universally resolve any ambiguity in favor of the patient and against the healthcare provider and organization or system.

The circumstances of a patient signing a consent form may also make the form suspect as substantive evidence of consent. If a patient presents a credible legal case that he or she was quickly handed a form and told to sign it at the height of an emergency and did not understand it, a court or jury may believe the patient and discount the form as evidence.

Finally, providers are warned never to fashion consent forms to limit or exclude provider liability for healthcare malpractice while the patient is under the provider's care. Such forms amount to *exculpatory contracts*, which courts generally find unconscionable and unacceptable in the healthcare delivery setting.

Documentation in the Patient Care Record

Documentation of informed consent to examination and intervention in a patient care record (typically during an initial patient visit) also may appear in short and long forms. The patient may or may not be asked to initial or sign the entry, attesting consent, in the record. Exhibit 4–5 is an example of long-form patient care record informed consent documentation.

Informed Consent Checklists or Standard Operating Procedures

Primary healthcare professionals can normally rely on abbreviated documentation of consent in patient care records when the healthcare organization or system has established either standard operating procedures for patient informed consent to specific procedures, or specialized informed consent checklists that the primary healthcare providers (not the patients) sign and date to verify that patient informed consent was obtained. Standard operating procedures or checklists outline all the required disclosure elements necessary to obtain patients' informed consent and should be retained at least until the state's statute of limitations for legal actions has expired.

A sample informed consent policy statement that might appear in a department quality management or policies and procedures manual might read as follows:

> This department and its primary and support healthcare and other professionals respect the autonomy right of all patients having legal and mental capacity (or valid surrogate decision-makers otherwise) to receive sufficient disclosure information about prospective examinations and recommended interventions so as to enable them to make knowing, informed choices about whether to accept or reject them. Such disclosure universally includes information related to the following:
>
> 1. The patient's health problem and the parameters of any proposed patient history and physical examination
>
> 2. Post-examination, the patient's evaluative findings and diagnosis, and information about the recommended intervention(s)
>
> 3. Material risks, if any, associated with the recommended intervention(s). (Material risks include important "decisional" risks [including foreseeable

complications possibly associated with the recommended intervention] or precautions that would cause an ordinary, reasonable patient to think carefully when deciding whether to undergo or reject the recommended intervention).

4. All reasonable alternatives, if any, to the proposed intervention(s) (i.e., other effective potential interventions that would be acceptable substitutes under legal standards of practice.) The provider must be sure to include discussion of the relative risks and benefits of alternative interventions.

5. Expected benefits, or goals, and prognosis associated with the recommended intervention(s).

After such disclosure of information is made, patient questions are actively solicited and answered to the patient's satisfaction by the primary healthcare professional, and examination and/or intervention does not proceed unless and until the patient formally assents to it/them.

Memoranda for Record

On an *ad hoc* basis, primary healthcare professionals may wish to create office memoranda that memorialize informed consent disclosure and patient assent for individual patients, which may or may not be filed in the patients' care records. Such memoranda are typically created for special cases (e.g., active litigation patients, or patients who express strong dissatisfaction with the department or facility/system offering care). Memoranda might be created in cases in which patient informed consent is not routinely individually documented in detail in patient care records, and where, in these special cases, detail about the informed consent process is deemed advisable.

MANAGED CARE INFORMED CONSENT DOCUMENTATION ISSUES

Managed care had created at least three special informed consent documentation issues, which bear mentioning here. First, there is a public perception—correct or incorrect—that managed care organizations have devised "gag clauses" in provider employment contracts that disallow employee-providers from disclosing to patients reasonable alternatives to recommended healthcare interventions not offered routinely within the organization or system. Such contractual provisions, to the extent that they exist, derogate from healthcare provider and organization respect for patient autonomy over healthcare decision-making, and are unethical in their application. Health professional codes of ethics and state and federal statutes and administrative regulations have largely made their usage nonexistent. Second, healthcare professionals whose compensation is variable, dependent on how much money they save their employing healthcare organizations, should disclose that fact to patients under their care, and should consider adding the following disclaimer (if true):

> I will not violate my special fiduciary duty of trust and fidelity owed to you as a patient, nor will I compromise the quality of your care, because I receive variable incentive pay from my employer for helping to contain healthcare costs.

The third and final point under managed care is that legal and health professional ethical duties incumbent upon primary healthcare providers have not changed significantly to accommodate the business of managed care. While it may seem to be a time burden to routinely make informed consent disclosure to patients (and to document it, when appropriate or required), it is imperative to do so out of respect for patient autonomy— the same autonomy right that each of us would wish respected were we the patient.

HIPAA INFORMED CONSENT ISSUES

Pursuant to the original regulations implementing the Health Insurance Portability and Accountability Act of 1996 (HIPAA), "covered" healthcare providers were to have been required to obtain patient informed consent in writing for use by the provider of the patient's protected health information (PHI) for treatment, operations, and reimbursement. However, by March 2002, then incoming, now former Health and Human Services Secretary Tommy Thompson wanted to review the HIPAA regulations to ensure they would not overburden business. The final federal rules published in November 2002 permitted, but did not require, covered entities to voluntarily obtain patient informed consent for utilization of their PHI for treatment, operations, and reimbursement for services. Providers and organizations, if they choose to obtain patient informed consent, are free to design any process that suits their needs.

Focus on Ethics

Research, compare, and contrast the informed consent ethical provisions from the following professional associations representing primary healthcare disciplines: the American Medical Association, the American Nurses Association, the American Occupational Therapy Association, and the American Physical Therapy Association. (Include your own discipline if distinct from those listed above.) Do all disciplines' ethics codes expressly address patient informed consent? Who is covered by the duty to obtain or ensure patient informed consent to intervention? Which discipline's informed consent provision is clearest in its language; which, in your opinion, is/are most reflective of health professional ethics codes' patient–public protective function? Share results and opinions.

CHAPTER SUMMARY

The law of informed consent may seem complicated; however, meeting legal and professional ethical standards for disclosure is not only mandatory but also relatively easy to do. Every primary healthcare provider, regardless of level of care or practice setting, is required by law to gain patients' informed consent to examination and intervention.

Although the elements of legally sufficient informed patient consent vary from state to state, there is a core checklist of typically required disclosure information. The checklist includes examination/evaluative findings, diagnosis, prognosis, and information about recommended and alternative interventions, including their relative material (decisional) risks and expected benefits. Patient (or surrogate decision-maker) questions must be actively solicited and satisfactorily answered. Providers must always remember to communicate this and all information to patients in a language (including sign) that patients understand, and at their level of understanding. Minimize the use of health professional jargon!

There are many acceptable formats for documenting that patient informed consent was obtained before examination and intervention. These range from reference to clinic, departmental, or organization/ system policies and procedures to detailed documentation on consent forms or in patient care records. Careful attention to the processes of documentation of patient informed consent serves simultaneously to improve the quality of patient care and to manage healthcare malpractice risk exposure in clinical practice.

NOTES AND REFERENCES

1. Two legal case decisions that derogate from this norm are: *Spence v. Todaro,* No. 943757 (E.D., Pa. 1994) (physical therapy) and *Friter & Friter v. Iolab Corp.*, 607 A.2d 1111 (Pa. Super. Ct., 1992) (clinical laboratory scientists), in which judges ruled that, under Pennsylvania law, patient informed consent is only required for surgical procedures.

2. The Patient Self-Determination Act, 42 U.S.C. Section1395cc(f) (1)(A)(i).

3. *Schloendorff v. Society of New York Hospital,* 105 N.E. 92 (N.Y. 1914).

4. *Natanson v. Kline,* 186 Kan. 393, 350 P.2d 1093 (1960).

5. *Canterbury v. Spence,* 464 F.2d 772 (D.C. Cir., 1972), cert. denied, 409 U.S. 1064 (1974). The term cert. denied, as used here, indicates that the U.S. Supreme Court refused, as a matter of discretion, to hear the case on appeal.

6. Hudson T. Informed consent problems become more complicated. *Hospitals.* 1991; 65:38–40.

7. Katz J. *The Silent World of Doctor and Patient.* New York: Free Press; 1986:85–103.

ADDITIONAL SUGGESTED READINGS AND NOTES

Code of Ethics for the Physical Therapist. Alexandria, VA: American Physical Therapy Association; 2010. On July 1, 2010, the American Physical Therapy Association's Ethics and Judicial Committee and Board of Directors replaced Principle 2.4A. ("A physical therapist shall respect the patient's/client's right to make decisions regarding the recommended plan of care, including consent, modification, or refusal.") with Principle 2C ("Physical therapists shall provide the information necessary to allow patients or their surrogates to make informed decisions about physical therapy care or participation in clinical research.").

Council on Ethical and Judicial Affairs: Ethical issues in managed care. *JAMA.* 1995; 273:330–335.

Kaplan M. Wie sagt man . . . ? sites that'll translate anything. *USA Weekend.* 1996; Oct. 8–10:16.

Landro L. Consent forms. *Wall Street Journal,* 2008; February 6: D1, 3. In this summary, Landro highlights "current events" in the law and ethics of patient informed consent. Informed consent may be the "biggest misnomer in medicine," because, according to Dr. Fay Rosovsky (see next reference below), many hospitals treat IC as an "administrative nuisance" rather than a means of respecting patient autonomy over care-related decision-making. New CMS guidelines include informed consent disclosure language similar to that described in this chapter, with inclusion of a provision describing the probable consequences of declining recommended or alternative therapies (informed refusal). The Joint Commission advocates a "teach back" method for obtaining patient informed consent, having patients repeat what they hear from their primary providers. The Veterans Administration's iMedConsent process utilizes electronic pictorial and word consent forms written at the 6th grade level to ensure comprehension by most or all patients of what is said to them, and to document their understanding. Finally, Landro illustrates a University of California at San Francisco study that demonstrated a significant increase in patient comprehension for informed consent forms written at the 6th grade level from 28% to 98%.

Rozovsky FA. *Consent to Treatment,* 3rd ed. Gaithersburg, MD: Aspen Publishers; 2001.

Scott RW. *Promoting Legal and Ethical Awareness: A Primer for Health Professionals and Patients.* St. Louis, MO: Mosby-Elsevier; 2009.

SDLFreeTranslation.com. Homepage (a free transcription Web site, medical translation assistance). Accessed June 30, 2011, from http://www.freetranslation.com

REVIEW CASE STUDIES

1. E, a physical therapist employed by ABC General Hospital, treats F, a female patient referred for "evaluation and treatment" for her complaint of right sternoclavicular pain. E examines patient F and decides to use myofascial mobilization techniques to release local adhesions. The intervention caused patient F some moderate discomfort, and E moderated his manual pressure over patient F's sternum each time she voiced any complaints of discomfort. At home that evening, patient F began to experience right breast

discomfort, and she and her husband discussed E's manual techniques. Angered by what they believed to have been a sexual battery, patient F and her husband file a complaint against ABC. How might this situation have been prevented?

Patient M is admitted to XYZ Rehabilitation Center for short-term stroke rehabilitation. Patient M displays mild aphasia; has moderate loss of function of his right (dominant) hand; and is brought to the facility in a wheelchair. As part of the admissions process, patient M's wife, N, is directed to read and sign the facility's standard consent/release form, which reads in part as follows:

I hereby agree to hold harmless ABC Rehabilitation Center and its agents, employees, and volunteers, for any injury suffered by me incident to my care, except that liability is not waived for acts or omissions amounting to gross negligence, recklessness, or intentional misconduct.

During the admission intake process, a volunteer transporting M by wheelchair runs his left leg into a door frame, fracturing it. Liability?

DISCUSSION: REVIEW CASE STUDIES

1. This complaint could have been prevented if E had taken the time to explain carefully to patient F his evaluative findings concerning her condition; the nature of myofascial mobilization; the risks and complications associated with it, such as soft tissue discomfort, erytherna, and perhaps mild bruising; and the viable alternatives to myofascial mobilization, such as heat, ice, and stretching, and postural exercises. E then should have shared literature about myofascial mobilization with patient F and solicited and answered her questions. At F's request, E also could have included patient F's husband in the discussion. E should have documented the processes used to obtain F's informed consent to examination and intervention. For procedures that bring a provider's hands in close proximity to a patient's private zones of contact, prudence would also dictate the offer of a chaperone of the same gender as the patient.

2. Patient M has an actionable cause of action for negligence against XYZ Rehabilitation Center. Hospitals are normally vicariously

liable for the negligence of their volunteers, who are treated as employees for the purpose of such a determination. The "consent/release" form that patient M's wife was required to sign on admission is an exculpatory contract that has no legal effect. Healthcare facilities cannot limit their liability for professional or ordinary negligence incident to healthcare activities through such an attempted waiver of liability. See *Tunkl v. Regents of the University of California*, 60 Cal. 2d 92 (1963). Depending on state law, the facility might have been able to require patient M to take a claim to some sort of alternative dispute resolution, such as arbitration, instead of filing a lawsuit. However, such an agreement should be made separate and apart from any consent forms a patient is asked to sign.

REVIEW ACTIVITY

Assume that you are a healthcare provider who is a HIPAA "covered entity" for compliance with HIPAA and its implementing regulations. Design a simple informed consent policy for disclosing to patients how their PHI will be used and disseminated in your practice.

CHAPTER 5

Patient Care Documentation and Clinical Quality-Risk Management Programs and Initiatives

This chapter examines the processes of patient care-related quality and liability risk management. While the concept of liability risk management is straightforward, *quality management* is a more global concept that includes development, implementation, monitoring, analysis, and revision, as needed, of information, liability-avoidance, patient care, and resource utilization healthcare delivery systems. Healthcare organizations, systems, and providers must carefully adhere to specific compliance requirements of accreditation and oversight entities, as applicable, to achieve and maintain accreditation, certification, and the capability to receive third-party payment for patient care services.

INTRODUCTION

The process of quality management of healthcare delivery is ever evolving. Once referred to as *quality assurance*, the systematic management of the quality of patient care delivery now goes by one of many labels including "quality improvement," "quality assessment and improvement," "continuous quality improvement," "total quality management," "promoting quality/managing risk," "improving organizational performance," and "performance improvement," among others. The change in emphasis in healthcare quality management is away from the impossible task of "assuring" quality to continuously striving to improve the quality of healthcare delivery.

The term *quality* is not easily defined. Its most important attribute is probably how the purchasers or users of goods and services (including patients and clients who receive health professional services, and their significant others) characterize the healthcare services and related products that they receive. In that respect, modern quality management is *customer-driven*. Quality, though, is more than just the consumer's perception of how "good" a supplier's product or service is.

It is also a reflection of how the professionals making the product or rendering the service feel, collectively and individually, about their work product. Quality is also the characterization of reputation and prestige afforded to one's work product by competitors, third-party payers, accreditation and oversight entities, and relevant others.

A comprehensive healthcare quality management program has, among others, the following characteristics:

1. It is patient-focused.

2. It requires top management commitment, vision, and leadership to be effective.

3. It requires a daily commitment by the entire organization/system to excellence and to continuous incremental improvement in the quality of patient care delivery.

4. It uses scientific and quantifiable methods to measure, evaluate, and improve processes of patient care delivery and patient care outcomes (evidence-based practice).

5. It empowers employees, working collectively in small multidisciplinary, cross-departmental teams, to proactively define and solve organizational problems and seek out opportunities for improvement of processes and outcomes of patient care.

6. It is based on a written plan of action.

7. It recognizes as normal the process variations along the continuum of quality patient care delivery.

8. It celebrates successes and rewards high quality performance.

9. It redirects the focus of error correction from individuals to processes and outcomes, and demands collective departmental and organizational responsibility both for successes and failures.

10. It requires ongoing, systematic training, education, and development.

11. It does not "settle" for minimally-acceptable patient care standards, processes, and outcomes. (Minimally acceptable quality patient care is a benchmark only for the legal standard of care, that is, for determining whether healthcare malpractice has occurred or not. It is an inappropriate standard for determining whether optimal quality patient care has been delivered.)

High quality patient care (including precise, comprehensive patient care documentation) literally means life versus death for patients on a daily basis. Orszac reported that, as a $2.6 trillion industry, healthcare in the United States is idle more than a quarter of the time (i.e., on weekends).[1] This fact is reflected in mortality statistics involving patients presenting to hospitals with myocardial infarction on weekends, where there are ten more patient deaths per 1,000 than during the Monday-to-Friday workweek. New York University's Langone Medical Center recently established relative intense quality monitoring standards on all of its physicians in order to improve patient quality outcomes.[1]

ACCREDITATION ENTITIES

There are three primary private accrediting organizations in the United States. Accreditation by these entities is carried out on a strictly voluntary basis. Substantial community and professional goodwill (reputation enhancement) can result from accreditation by one or more of these organizations.

The Joint Commission—formerly the Joint Commission on Accreditation of Healthcare Organizations—is a Chicago-based private organization that accredits hospitals, ambulatory care and surgery centers, laboratories, long-term care facilities, home health agencies, assisted living centers, and behavioral healthcare organizations across the United States and internationally. Accreditation by the Joint Commission, as with the other nongovernmental entities, is voluntary.

The Joint Commission's focus for hospitals is performance improvement, or improving organizational performance. It has a dual focus on processes and outcomes of patient-care service delivery. Its elements of performance, or performance measures (formerly "indicators"), are standards used to evaluate healthcare organizations undergoing accreditation. Hospitals and departments typically monitor major performance measures on an ongoing basis, with the principal foci on patient care and safety measures, including, among others, two-way communications between patients and healthcare providers, delivery of medications, security, and wound care.

Sentinel events—unanticipated occurrences that result in serious bodily harm or death to patients—are always intensively and immediately responded to and investigated, within the responsible facility and by outside entities, including private accreditation bodies and governmental oversight agencies, such as the Food and Drug Administration (for injuries or deaths from defective medical products) and the Department of Health and Human Services.

One evaluative model for performance assessment is FMEA (failure mode and effect analysis). This quality management tool is a systematic procedure utilized to rank and prioritize possible causes of product failure and implement preventive measures. As a quality insurance (QI) process, it was originally adapted by automobile manufacturers from engineering in the 1960s. FMEA involves intensive analysis of the component parts of a process with the goal of preventing product failure. Data and documentation about processes are crucial for its successful implementation. Like total quality management (TQM) in the past, FMEA is currently being applied to health service delivery. TQM is based in large part on the industrial model developed by W. Edward Deming, PhD, who consulted with and helped revitalize Japanese industry after World War II.

In its annual *Comprehensive Accreditation Manual for Hospitals*, the Joint Commission addresses patient care documentation processes and standards in its Patient-Centered Communication Standards and Elements of Performance chapter.

Focus on Ethics

Access the Joint Commission's Web site (http://www.jointcommission .org). Under the accreditation and hospitals tabs, peruse the Patient-Centered Communication Standards and Elements of Performance. Cross-check the contents for medical records standards contained in RC.02.01.01 with those in place in your hospital, clinic, organization, or system. Ascertain that you and your colleagues meet the ethics-based performance expectations for respecting patients' rights contained in RI.01.01.01.

CARF International, formerly the Commission on Accreditation of Rehabilitation Facilities, a Tucson, Arizona-based private organization, accredits 47,000 programs and services worldwide. The services it accredits include: aging services, behavioral health (including opioid treatment programs), business and services management networks, child and youth services, employment and community services (including vision rehabilitation), and medical rehabilitation (including durable medical equipment, prosthetics, and orthotics and supplies). Its definition of quality service is that it is individualized to particular patient needs, responsive, and team-based.

The National Committee for Quality Assurance (NCQA), founded in 1990, is a Washington, DC–based nonprofit private 501(c)(3) organization that accredits health plans and organizations that cover 109 million people in the United States (comprising 70.5% of Americans enrolled in health plans). Its defines quality in terms of accountability, transparency, and value, and advocates a four-step method for quality improvement: assessment, planning, implementation and evaluation. It uses the independently audited Health Plan Employer Data and Information Set (HEDIS) to measure and report on healthcare organization performance in 71 measures across 8 domains of care delivery. Its 2010 *State of Health Care Quality* examined the relationships between and among quality healthcare, the rising costs of healthcare delivery, and the effects of the economic downturn. (The report may be downloaded free-of-charge from the Web site.) NCQA cosponsors a Master of Science in Health Care Quality with George Washington University.

COMPONENTS OF A HEALTHCARE QUALITY MANAGEMENT PROGRAM

A comprehensive healthcare quality management program consists of at least the following component parts:

- Patient care process and outcome measurement, evaluation, and remediation activities
- Patient care documentation and healthcare information management
- Credentialing, privileging, and/or competency assessment activities involving all healthcare providers
- Resource utilization management
- Liability risk management activities

Patient Care Outcome Measurement, Evaluation, and Remediation Activities

Patient care process and outcome measurement, evaluation, and remediation activities encompass the systematic analysis of selected clinical indicators concerning important recurrent aspects of patient care. Patient care process and outcome measurement, evaluation, and remediation activities track patient–healthcare provider professional interactions along a continuum from advertising services, appointments, and intake, through examination, evaluation, formulation of diagnoses and prognoses, intervention, patient/family/significant other education, discharge, postdischarge activities, and follow-up, in every conceivable patient care setting, from hospital, to outpatient, to long-term care, to a patient home environment, among others. To concentrate improvement efforts where they will have the most effect, patient care process and outcome measurement, evaluation, and remediation activities focus on patient care activities that are high risk, high volume, or problem prone. In order to assess the efficacy of remedial interventions implemented by decision-makers, these systematic processes include a feedback loop to monitor success and to modulate or replace remedial interventions, as needed.

Patient Care Documentation and Health Information Management

The fundamental premise of the book is that documentation of patient care activities—whether reduced to writing on paper, or generated and stored electronically—is as important as the rendition of patient care itself. For the protection of patients, healthcare professionals, and healthcare delivery systems, substantial attention is directed toward providers' and systems' ethical and legal duties owed to patients under their care.

Documentation of care-related activities has lifelong importance to the patient, who depends on an accurate, clear, timely, thorough historical record of his or her health status, for current and future healthcare needs. It is equally important to the individual healthcare providers and healthcare organizations, for whom the patient care record memorializes the nature and quality of care rendered to the patient.

Documentation of patient care is crucial to the survival of a healthcare organization, because it forms the basis for third-party reimbursement and, in the form of a patient health record, serves as a business record, admissible in court as evidence of the nature and quality of patient care rendered in the facility. Documentation in a facility's quality management program also serves as evidence of compliance with laws, regulations, and accreditation standards, and helps prevent imposition of corporate liability against an organization or system for failing to monitor the quality of patient care rendered within the organization or system, and for failing to effectively maximize patient, visitor, and staff safety in its facilities, among other nondelegable duties. Finally, patient care documentation serves important societal interests, including use in clinical research on disease and injury.

Provider Credentialing, Privileging, and Competency Assessment Activities

For a variety of reasons, healthcare organizations need to assess the competence and character of their healthcare providers, support staff, and others working in their facilities. Healthcare facilities owe a special duty of care to patients cared for within their facilities, and are vicariously, or indirectly, liable for the negligence and other wrongful acts of employees acting within the scope of their employment. Under the legal theory of *corporate liability*, healthcare organizations are also primarily liable to patients for failure to monitor the competence of professional and support personnel, whether the patient care is rendered by employees or independent contractors.

Along with credentials privileging processes, healthcare organizations are responsible for ensuring the continuing competence of all of their staff. Included under this responsibility are training, continuing education, and cardiopulmonary resuscitation certification and recertification (as appropriate), among other activities.

Resource Utilization Management

In the current cost-containment-focused healthcare environment, the effective management of healthcare resources—human and nonhuman—is critical to a healthcare organization's or system's survival. Important areas of concern for resource and clinical managers include equitable patient access to available services, and length of care and post-discharge care, among others.

Liability Risk Management Activities

Liability risk management encompasses a wide range of variegated activities, including the following, in addition to striving toward optimal quality health professional service delivery:

- Patient, visitor, and staff safety activities
- Patient, visitor, staff, and public injury prevention, reporting, and investigation
- Infection control and waste management
- Calibration, maintenance, and replacement of equipment
- Patient satisfaction surveys

Liability risk management is an integral part of an overall quality management program. It shares similarities with other component activities, such as the patient care outcome measurement, evaluation, and remediation function, but is also characterized by fundamental differences that distinguish it from other quality management activities.

In terms of similarities to other quality management activities, liability risk management processes employ a similar methodology, including the identification of important aspects of care, development of measurement indicators that are examined on an ongoing basis, the systematic reporting of results, and the correction of identified problems. As with all other quality management activities, liability risk management processes have the effect of continuously improving and optimizing quality patient care delivery within facilities, organizations, and systems, and among individuals and practice groups.

Liability risk management activities differ, however, from the other quality management program components in several key respects. The focus of risk management activities is a *legal* rather than a patient-oriented focus. The principal purpose of risk management activities is to protect the facility and its providers by preventing or minimizing financial losses from legal actions arising from patient care or other activities conducted in the facility. Although risk management activities tend to promote optimal quality patient care, their focus is on "minimally acceptable standards of clinical practice," that is, the legal standard of care—the legal benchmark in malpractice actions delineating negligent and nonnegligent patient care. Risk management activities also differ from the other component quality management activities with regard to their sphere of participant inclusiveness. Patient care process and outcome measurement, evaluation, and remediation, credentialing and competency assessment, and resource utilization management are all internal processes that involve primarily healthcare clinicians and administrators, whereas risk management activities include professionals outside of healthcare delivery and administration, particularly in-house and consulting legal counsel, along with judges, juries, and other judicial system professionals.

Of particular interest to healthcare facility risk managers is the management of potentially compensable events, involving adverse outcomes of patient care and alleged or actual injuries or other adverse events. Risk managers are also responsible for managing claims against the organization, and potential and pendent legal and administrative actions. Risk management, however, is more than just reactive in nature. Risk managers attempt to prevent potentially compensable events from arising through such processes as occurrence screening of potential risk situations. These situations include facility-incurred trauma, complications, and infection; unplanned return patient visits or surgery; unscheduled readmissions within a specified time period after a prior admission; and unfavorable trends in patient satisfaction surveys. (Since 2008, Medicare, and subsequently other third-party payers, have refused to reimburse hospitals for select serious adverse events [called *never events*].)

CONFIDENTIALITY CONSIDERATIONS IN PATIENT CARE QUALITY MANAGEMENT

Quality assurance/improvement documents normally enjoy a degree of protection from disclosure or release to patients, their attorneys, and others, under statutory and/or common law. Different rules may apply to patient care and related documentation maintained by healthcare organizations primarily governed under federal or state law, or both.

Under common law, quality management-related documentation enjoys qualified protection either because it is classified as *self-evaluative* material, whose purpose is to improve the quality of patient care delivery now or in the future or, in the case of incident reporting documentation, because it is prepared at the direction of a healthcare facility attorney or other official in anticipation of litigation and falls under "attorney–client privilege."

So that no question can arise about whether documentation is in fact quality management–related documentation, organization and department quality and risk managers should ensure that such documents are prominently labeled as "quality assurance," "quality improvement," or "quality management" documentation (as appropriate under individual state law), and display the warning that such documentation is not for release to third parties.

RISK MANAGEMENT PATIENT CARE RECORD REVIEW

One of the most interesting duties of a healthcare organization risk manager is to conduct a patient care record review, on request, for an attorney preparing to defend the facility against a malpractice or other legal action. This review is critically important to the defense of a claim or lawsuit and must be performed in a systematic, accurate, objective, thorough, and concise manner. The reviewer should ask the attorney requesting the review to provide a copy of the patient-plaintiff 's complaint, so that the reviewer is familiar with the patient's precise allegations against the healthcare organization and/or its providers.

The risk manager conducting a litigation record review must remain impartial and report, first orally, then, if directed by counsel, produce a report that is free of bias if it is to be useful to legal counsel. Attorneys generally prefer that a record review report be summarized chronologically and that it contain appropriate headings and subheadings. Many attorneys do not mind, and some even expect, the candid opinions of the reviewer concerning potential liability and damages (extent of injury) issues.

Risk managers analyzing patient care records for possible litigation must be sure, when writing up their reports, to label the work product (from first draft to final report) as "attorney–client work product, prepared for, and at the direction of, the facility attorney in anticipation of and in preparation for litigation." This disclaimer (or similar language, according to individual state law) maximizes the likelihood that the report is protected from disclosure to a patient-plaintiff 's attorney under pretrial discovery rules.

Exhibit 5–1 presents an example of an outline format for a patient care record review litigation report.

Exhibit 5–1 Example of a Risk Management Treatment Record Review Report Format

XYZ General Hospital
Anytown, USA

Risk Management Patient Treatment Record Review Report

1. Patient's name: _____

2. Admission (or treatment) date(s): _____

3. Admission (treatment) diagnoses: _____

4. Clinical resume (chronological): _____

5. Summary of patient allegation(s): _____

6. Synopsis of investigation/interviews: _____

7. Analysis of liabilities: _____

8. Damages (injury) assessment: _____

9. Other information and issues: _____

10. "Attorney-client work product, prepared for and at the direction of the facility attorney in anticipation of and in preparation for litigation."

Signature block and title of reviewer

Date report submitted

MONITORING INFORMED CONSENT AS A QUALITY IMPROVEMENT INDICATOR

An area of special concern and confusion for many healthcare providers is patient informed consent to examination and intervention. This is a complicated area of healthcare malpractice law, often characterized by state-specific statutory and common law disclosure elements that must be imparted to patients, as well as a wide range of potential documentation formats to memorialize informed consent processes.

More and more, healthcare providers who obtain patient informed consent to examination and intervention on a recurring basis are utilizing audiovisual aids to educate patients about processes and options. These supplements or alternatives to consent forms can take the form of descriptive pamphlets, individual or small group classes, audio and videotape presentations, and computer-generated passive and interactive presentations. These kinds of presentation formats for informed consent information enhance primary healthcare provider–patient communication and patient comprehension, and set the stage for focused discussion after the presentation on specific patient concerns.

As a supplement to or substitute for consent forms as the standard means of documenting patient informed consent, many providers and organizations or systems are employing review questionnaires, completed either on paper or on computer, to ensure that patients truly understand the material risks and benefits of and alternatives to proposed interventions. The Veterans Administration's IMed Consent system utilizes diagrams, pictures, and other elementary education tools to communicate with patients, and their informed consent to medical and surgical interventions.[2] Similar innovative models are in place in medical centers and clinics across the United States, Canada, and Europe.

Primary healthcare professionals from every healthcare discipline should consider developing patient educational programs about recurring procedures and therapeutic interventions, and supplement them with appropriate audiovisual aids. Review questionnaires also should be developed to ensure that patients understand what they are "consenting" to. These processes and documents serve to memorialize the informed consent process and may be admissible evidence of what was said to and done for a patient during informed consent disclosure.

Providers should consider monitoring informed consent disclosure, including HIPAA informed consent procedures, as part of quality and risk management programs in their organizations. A sample measure for informed consent might be, "Patients will give informed consent before examination or intervention commences." Such a measure can be monitored through patient record review of informed consent documentation, direct observation of audiovisual patient education informed consent programs, and discussion with selected patients about their contents, administration of questionnaires or quizzes to patients after informed consent disclosure, and general patient interviews. An example of a generic informed consent patient questionnaire appears in **Exhibit 5–2**.

Exhibit 5–2 Example of a Generic Informed Consent Patient Questionnaire

Please answer the following questions to the best of your ability. Your answers and comments will be kept strictly confidential.

1. What health problem are you being treated for?

2. What is your healthcare provider's name?

3. Did your healthcare provider obtain your informed consent to treatment?

(If "no," skip to Question 9.)

4. What treatment did your healthcare provider recommend for your condition?

5. What benefits would this treatment offer?

6. Are there serious risks associated with the proposed treatment? If so, what are they?

7. Are there any other treatment options for your condition? If so, what are they?

8. Did your healthcare provider use audiovisual aids (e.g., pamphlets, videos) to help explain your condition and/or treatment? If so, what kinds of audiovisual aids were used? Were they helpful to you in making your decision about treatment?

9. Did you ask any questions about your treatment before accepting it? (Please indicate if you declined treatment.)

10. Were you satisfied with your provider's explanation of your condition and treatment options? Did you feel like you were in control of the decision-making process?

11. Please feel free to offer any other comments or make suggestions for improving our service. Thank you for taking the time to complete this questionnaire.

CHAPTER SUMMARY

Every healthcare organization has a primary legal duty to direct and oversee patient care delivery and promote optimal patient, visitor, and staff safety in the facility. This is carried out through a formal, systematic, comprehensive quality management program. Quality management encompasses patient care process and outcome measurement and evaluation activities, such as peer review and clinical indicator studies; staff credentialing/privileging and competency review activities; resource utilization management; patient care documentation, and health information and liability risk management activities.

Although the "buzz words"—quality assurance, quality improvement, continuous quality improvement, total quality management, improving organizational performance, the Deming method, and FMEA, among others—may be accreditation entity–specific and evolve over time, the basic premise remains the same: to provide optimal quality patient care and to protect healthcare providers, organizations, and systems from unwarranted liability exposure and losses. Quality management activities are coordinated at the organization and department levels by quality improvement coordinators. An optimally effective quality management program is patient-focused, guided, and strongly supported by top management, and empowering of individual entrepreneurs at the lowest operational levels, who are best equipped to suggest opportunities both to improve patient care and to minimize risk.

NOTES AND REFERENCES

The general outline of a model healthcare quality/risk management program presented in this section is not intended to replicate any particular program of any organization, system, professional association, or accreditation entity. The concepts presented are generic in nature, although the model program is intended to be comprehensive.

1. Orszac P. Health Care's Lost Weekend. *New York Times.* 2010; Oct. 4:A23.
2. http://www1.va.gov/vehuVeterans Administration's eHealth University. Class #154 (provides programmed instruction that overviews the VA's IMed informed consent processes for providers, free of charge). Accessed June 30, 2011, from http://www1.va.gov/vehu

ADDITIONAL SUGGESTED READINGS

Beranova E, Sykes C. A systematic review of computer-based softwares for educating patients with coronary artery disease. 2007; 66(1): 21–28.

Berwick DM. Continuous improvement as an ideal in health care. *New England Journal of Medicine.* 1989; 320:53–56.

CARF (Commission on Accreditation of Rehabilitation Facilities). Homepage. Accessed July 1, 2011, from http://www.carf.org

Gilles A. *Improving the Quality of Patient Care.* Hoboken, NJ: John Wiley & Sons; 1997.

Hutson MM, Blaha JD. Patients' recall of preoperative instruction for informed consent for an operation. *Journal of Bone and Joint Surgery.* 1991; 73-A:160–162.

The Joint Commission. *Comprehensive Accreditation Manual for Hospitals* (current edition). Accessed June 30, 2011, from http://www.jcrinc.com/Accreditation-Manuals/PCAH11/2130/

The Joint Commission. Homepage. Accessed July 1, 2011, from http://www.jointcommission.org

Malecki MS. RM's careful review of record can be a boost to hospital's attorney. *Hospital Risk Management.* 1991; March: 1–3.

McDermott RE, Mikulak RJ, Beauregard MR. *The Basics of FMEA.* London: Kraus Organization Ltd; 1996.

Muir J. The quest for quality. *PT Magazine.* 2004; 12:7.

National Committee for Quality Assurance (NCQA). Homepage. Accessed July 1, 2011, from http://www.ncqa.org

National Committee for Quality Assurance (NCQA). *State of Health Care Quality.* Washington, DC: HCQA; 2004.

New York University (NYU) Langone Medical Center. Homepage. Accessed July 1, 2011, from http://www.med.nyu.edu

Pettus MC. *The Savvy Patient: The Ultimate Advocate for Quality Health Care.* Richmond, VA: Capital City Books; 2004.

Shojania KG, Grimshaw JM. Evidence-based quality improvement: The state of the science. *Health Affairs.* 2005; 24(1):138–150.

Walton M. *The Deming Management Method.* New York, NY: Perigee Books; 1986.

Winslow R. Videos, questionnaires aim to expand role of patients in treatment decisions. *Wall Street Journal.* 1992; February 25: B1, B6.

Woodruff W. The confidentiality of medical quality assurance records. *Army Lawyer.* 1987; May:5.

REVIEW ACTIVITIES

1. Review the American Physical Therapy Association's Defensive Documentation for Patient/Client management at their Web site, http://www.apta.org. Compare and contrast similar risk management-focused patient care documentation guidelines promulgated by other rehabilitation professional associations and groups.

2. Design an instrument to measure healthcare provider voluntary compliance with HIPAA informed consent for utilization of PHI within your organization.

3. Design a five question, multiple choice review quiz for patients undergoing a recurrent intervention carried out in your clinic, covering the substantive aspects of the procedure that the patients should be aware of before agreeing to its use on them. Implement the quiz as a means of assessing provider–patient communication during informed consent processes.

5-A

Example of a Peer Review Work Sheet for the Evaluation of Interdisciplinary Primary Healthcare Professionals in a Rehabilitation Setting

ABC Rehabilitation Center

Peer Record Review Work Sheet

Patient's Name _____

Inpatient?   Y   N

Current status:

_____ Undergoing rehabilitation

_____ Discharged with in-clinic intervention

_____ Discharged to: (home, long-term care facility, etc.)

_____ Discharged secondary to nonattendance

_____ Other (specify): _____

Primary healthcare provider's name: _____

1. Are initial examination, progress, and discharge notes written in the appropriate format? (If "no," specify the deficiencies noted.)   Y   N

2. Are objective findings (e.g., for range of motion, muscle strength, girths) written in quantitative terms, whenever possible?

   Y   N

3. Are evaluative findings and diagnoses based on documented objective findings?   Y   N

4. (When applicable) Does the plan of care include or address any specific intervention requested or ordered by a referring physician?   Y   N

5. Are patient care goals reflective of patient needs and desires, and written in quantitative terms, with time frames for their achievement?   Y   N

6. In the reviewer's opinion, were patient care activities adequately documented? (If not, explain)   Y   N

7. Additional reviewer comments:

Reviewer's Signature and Stamp   Date of Review

Sample Patient Satisfaction Survey

ABC Rehabilitation Center

Patient Satisfaction Survey
Please help us improve our service to you and others by answering the following questions and then depositing the anonymous survey in the survey box in the patient dressing rooms. Thank you for your input.

1. Please rate our service overall: Excellent   Good   Fair   Poor

2. How would you rate the following?

   Check-in time: Excellent   Good   Fair   Poor
   Timeliness of being seen by
   therapist: Excellent   Good   Fair   Poor

3. How would you rate the attitudes of our staff?

   Receptionist: Excellent   Good   Fair   Poor
   Therapist: Excellent   Good   Fair   Poor
   Assistant and/or aide/volun-
   teer (please specify which):   Excellent   Good   Fair   Poor

   Comments (optional):

4. If any members of our staff were particularly helpful to you, please let us know so we may recognize them and show our appreciation.

5. In your own words, what did you learn about managing your condition or problem?

Thank you again for your comments.
Rehab Staff and Management

CHAPTER 6

Current Issues in Patient Care Documentation

This chapter presents a summary of selected important patient care documentation issues that providers encounter in clinical practice. The areas addressed include: advance directives and the Patient Self-Determination Act; adverse incident documentation issues; clinical practice standards and guidelines as evidence of the legal standard of care; documenting the care of sexual assault patients; documenting the use of physical restraints; electronic health records (EHRs); HIPAA; legal issues associated with reimbursement documentation; mandatory reporting requirements, including child, spouse, and elder abuse, occupational and communicable diseases, and defective medical devices; patient discharge documentation; patient noncompliance, disengagement, and abandonment; withdrawal of life support/DNR guidelines; and telehealth documentation issues.

ADVANCE DIRECTIVES AND THE PATIENT SELF-DETERMINATION ACT

The Patient Self-Determination Act[1] (hereinafter "Act"), signed into law by former President Bush in November 1990, codifies a patient's common law right to control healthcare decisions—both routine and extraordinary. When it became effective on December 1, 1991, the Act bound hospitals, health maintenance organizations, long-term care facilities, hospices, and other healthcare entities participating in Medicare and Medicaid to its provisions.

The fundamental purpose of the Act is to ensure that providers and healthcare organizations provide patient education about informed consent and the right of patients to make advance directives. *Advance directives* include legal instruments such as the *living will,*[2] *durable power of attorney for healthcare decision-making,*[3] *out-of-facility do not resuscitate order,*[4] *and declaration for mental health treatment,*[5] which memorialize patient desires concerning life-sustaining measures to be taken and decision making should the patient subsequently become legally incapacitated.

A key concept underlying the Act is respect for a patient's right to give informed consent to health-related examination and intervention. Under this process, a healthcare provider must provide the patient with relevant disclosure information about a proposed examination or intervention to allow the patient to analyze the options and make an informed choice about whether to accept or reject examination or a recommended intervention (or insist on another reasonable alternative intervention—even under managed care).

Although the Act does not create any new substantive patient rights, it does impose burdensome procedural obligations on healthcare organizations and providers covered by the law. Among other requirements, the Act requires a covered healthcare provider or facility to do the following:

(1)

    (A) Provide written information (to patients) concerning:

        (i) An individual's rights under state law (whether statutory or as recognized by the courts of the state) to make decisions concerning . . . medical care, including the right to accept or refuse medical or surgical treatment and the right to formulate advance directives . . . and

        (ii) The written policies of the provider or organization respecting the implementation of such rights. . . .

    (B) Document in the individual's medical record whether or not the individual has executed an advance directive. . . .

  (2) The written information described in paragraph (1)(A) shall be provided to an adult individual:

    (A) In the case of a hospital, at the time of the individual's admission as an inpatient

    (B) In the case of a skilled nursing facility, at the time of the individual's admission as a resident

(C) In the case of a home health agency, in advance of the individual coming under the care of the agency.

Before any substantive care is undertaken, then, in any patient care setting, a patient must receive written information about the right to make informed decisions regarding examination and intervention and the right (consistent with state law) to make advance directives regarding future care in the event of the patient's incapacitation. Also, a covered healthcare facility must provide the patient with a written copy of the facility's policy on implementing the requirements of the Act.

In addition to its disclosure obligations discussed above, a healthcare organization covered by the Act has documentation responsibilities as well. The facility must annotate in a patient's care record whether the patient has signed an advance directive regarding future care.

The four relevant questions that a facility must ask of patients are the following:

1. Do you have any advance directives? If so, what kind?

2. Do you have a copy of your directives?

3. Have there been any changes to your directives? If so, what are they, and do you have documentation of the changes?

4. If not readily available, who can we contact to obtain them, and include them in your patient care records?

Larsen and Eaton carried out an exhaustive study of the Act and reported[6] that it has been relatively unsuccessful in safeguarding the rights of patients to make, and to have enforced, advance directives concerning health care. The reasons cited for the lack of success of the Act include the following:

- Lack of individual awareness on the part of primary healthcare professionals of the existence of the Act
- Reluctance on the part of patients and long-term care facility residents to execute advance directives
- Recalcitrance on the part of healthcare providers and organizations to honor valid advance patient directives, in part because they substitute their own values for those of patients or fear liability exposure.

Focus on Ethics

If you work in, or are affiliated with, a healthcare organization that utilizes patient advance directives as part of comprehensive patient care documentation, examine and evaluate the organization's policies and procedures related to their use. Answer the following specific queries.

1. How are relevant healthcare professionals (medical doctors, nurses, occupational and physical therapists, among others) made aware of existing patient advance directives?

2. How are patient advance directives displayed in patients' medical records?

3. What procedures, if any, are in place within the organization to assist patients who wish to make or modify existing advance directives?

4. Interview a select sample of relevant primary and support professionals about their attitudes toward patient advance directives. Do they share Larsen and Eaton's[6] concerns about advance directives and their use? If so, consider raising any issues that arise with the organization's quality management and/or institutional ethics committees?

ADVERSE INCIDENT DOCUMENTATION ISSUES

The incident report is used by healthcare clinicians, clinical managers, quality and risk management coordinators, organization and system administrators, and corporate attorneys to document and report adverse events that may have adverse legal and/or quality management implications for the healthcare organization/system and its providers. Incident reports are used to document adverse events involving patients, visitors, staff, or any other persons—including trespassers and others who may be on facility property without authorization.

Documentation of adverse incidents serves two main purposes. First, by reporting a suspected or actual injury or highlighting a safety concern, the incident report serves to alert management of a potential problem that may warrant corrective action. Thus, the incident report serves as a basis for continuous quality improvement in the facility. Second, the incident report memorializes important facts about an alleged incident that create a record for use in further investigation, in the event that a legal action results from the incident. In this respect, the incident report protects facility and healthcare provider business and legal interests.

Even with facility guidelines or statutory requirements in effect, healthcare providers "on the front line" may be confused about when to generate an incident report. Because incident reports are confidential, no incident should be considered too minor to report. At the other end of the scale, major incidents that involve police or firefighter intervention also require a facility incident report, in addition to any official police or fire report that might be generated.

Regarding the contents of an incident report form, the following should be included:

- *Administrative data* about the patient or other subject of the report, including, at a minimum, name and address, date of birth, gender, incident dates, and status (inpatient, outpatient, emergency, staff, visitor, etc.)
- *Patient diagnosis* and a brief summary of care rendered to the patient (Note: If the incident involves someone other than a patient, then the information required for patients would not be completed.)
- *Type of incident* (e.g., premises [e.g., wet floor], equipment, medication, exercise, modality, wound debridement, surgery, etc.)
- *Condition of person affected* after the occurrence: no apparent injury, minor injury, major injury, death
- *Course of action undertaken*
- *Witnesses*, if any
- *Description of the event.* All facility staff must receive training from the facility risk manager about how to write an incident report. This summary of an adverse event must:

   1. Be concise, yet thorough

2. Document objectively what was observed firsthand by the writer of the report (the percipient witness)

3. Delineate in quotes second-hand (hearsay) statements attributable to another person

4. Not contain any speculation as to the possible cause of an occurrence or injury

- *Typed or printed name and title and signature of the writer* of the report
- *Date report completed and date submitted* to the facility risk manager

An incident report also should be identified either as a "confidential quality assurance/quality improvement report" or as a "document prepared at the direction of the facility attorney in anticipation of or in preparation for litigation," according to applicable state or federal legal requirements. The specific language to be used should be decided by the facility attorney, administrators, and risk managers, because, in some jurisdictions, one designation (i.e., quality improvement or litigation) may afford greater confidentiality than the other. Under federal law and the law of many states, for example, quality improvement documentation may be virtually immune from disclosure to third parties, whereas documents prepared for litigation may enjoy only qualified immunity and may be subject to release to a patient-plaintiff if the document is essential to the plaintiff's case and the information contained therein cannot be obtained through any other means.

Even within major health systems, incident reports are sometimes labeled only as confidential. The label *confidential* normally does nothing to provide legal immunity from release. The term *confidential* merely pre-identifies a document as sensitive. The fact that such important reports are often mislabeled reinforces the need to include attorney-advisors in drafting and approving their implementation, and monitoring their use, as a means to minimize adverse legal consequences of patient care.

When an adverse incident involving patient injury occurs, a provider should also document concisely and objectively in the patient care record a summary of patient injury and intervention to aid the victim. Do not mention the incident report in the concomitant patient care record entry. An example of an incident report appears as **Exhibit 6–1**. A hypothetical problem involving incident reporting is presented in the review case studies section at the end of the chapter.

Exhibit 6–1 Example of an Incident Report

Quality Assurance Risk Management Report

WARNING: The information contained in this quality assurance document is confidential and subject to privilege under applicable state and federal law. Penalties may apply for unauthorized release. Do not file or refer to this document in any patient treatment record.

1. (Date/Time/Location of Incident)

_____

2. (Name/Age/Gender of Person[s] Involved)

_____

3. (If Incident Involved a Patient, State Patient's Principal Diagnosis and Name[s] of Attending Physician[s])

_____

4. (Description of Event)

_____

5. (Condition of Patient and/or Other Persons Affected, After Occurrence)

_____

6. (Name[s], Address[es], Phone Number[s] of Witness[es], if Any, and Each Witness's Description of Event)

_____

7. (Brief Description of Treatment Rendered, if Any)

_____

8. (Name, Title, and Position of Person Completing Form)

_____

9. (Signature of Preparer and Date of Report)

_____

Note to Preparer of Report: Forward through department of service chief to facility risk manager within 24 hours. Notify risk manager telephonically of event immediately after emergency, if any, is resolved.

CLINICAL PRACTICE GUIDELINES AS EVIDENCE OF THE LEGAL STANDARD OF CARE

In addition to expert testimony on the legal standard of care, many healthcare malpractice attorneys are turning to clinical practice guidelines and protocols to establish required practice standards in legal cases. These guidelines can take the form of federal or state statutory or regulatory requirements, professional association and accreditation standards, and healthcare organization internal policies, protocols, and procedures.

Often, patient and defense attorneys turn first to internal facility policy and procedures manuals for information on standards of practice in effect in the facility. Providers in the facility are presumed to know and to follow guidelines established in these protocols. If a provider fails to conform to procedures outlined in a protocol, then that fact alone may constitute substantial evidence that the provider breached the required standard of care.

For that reason, facilities and clinics that utilize practice guidelines should exercise restraint not to make the protocols too rigid, to the extent possible. For example, in physical therapy, there are many acceptable ways to care for a patient with adhesive capsulitis of the shoulder, including modalities, stretching, active assist, active, and resistive exercise, passive mobilization, and muscle energy techniques, among others. To limit physical therapists in a clinic to one or two of the above may needlessly create a practice standard that is higher than what the law requires. Wherever possible, a practice standard should contain a clause that allows professional healthcare clinicians the option of deviating from the standard in individual cases, based on their professional judgment.

The federal and state governments are exploring the use of practice guidelines to establish presumptive or conclusive compliance with legal standards of care as a method of malpractice tort reform. The federal Agency for Health Care Research and Quality (AHRQ), an agency of the Public Health Service, issued some 19 popular clinical practice guidelines between 1992 and 1996; however, the Agency ceased such issuance of guidelines due, in part, to their unintended use by attorneys in healthcare malpractice legal proceedings as evidence of the legal standard of care.

DOCUMENTING THE CARE OF SEXUAL ASSAULT PATIENTS

The interview, examination, and care of sexual assault or battery victims requires careful coordination of healthcare and law enforcement personnel. Not only must the patient's immediate and short-term physical and psychological needs be attended to, but important physical and testimonial evidence must be obtained and safeguarded in the patient's legal best interests (i.e., for successful subsequent prosecution of the offender).

Often, a patient who is the victim of a sexual assault will be treated under emergency circumstances, and her or his care will require the intervention of a designated sexual assault crisis team. Carefully drafted written policies governing the treatment of sexual assault victims is crucial to minimize additional trauma to the patient, and to collect, store, and transfer evidence to law enforcement authorities.

Before carrying out examination and initial treatment of a sexual assault victim, it is important to obtain the patient's informed consent. Depending on the patient's mental status, it may not be feasible to obtain the informed consent in a signed writing. In this case, a member of the crisis team witnessing the informed consent process should summarize the disclosure in the patient's initial examination and intervention documentation.

It is critically important that the examining physician expeditiously record his or her evaluative findings in the patient's emergency medical record. Any statements made by the patient should be included in this documentation and enclosed in quotes. This kind of *hearsay* evidence may be admissible in a legal proceeding as an "excited utterance" or "statement [made] for purposes of medical diagnosis or treatment."[7] Records of sexual assault victims should be maintained separate from general patient care records in a designated special handling file to safeguard the confidentiality of sensitive patient information and to ensure the medicolegal integrity of these records.

Another important issue is chain of custody of laboratory specimens and physical evidence obtained from the victim. Forensic specimens should be appropriately labeled on chain of custody documents after they are obtained by the examining physician and should be safeguarded under lock and key until they are transferred to law enforcement officials having jurisdiction over the criminal case. Patient specimens that are to be used for patient treatment do not normally require the special labeling and handling required for forensic specimens.

In November 2009, a CBS investigation revealed that of the 90,000 reported rapes in 2008, 20,000 rape kits lay languishing in police evidence lockers across the United States. These evidence kits were never sent to labs for testing, due in large part to the $1,500 cost of testing per kit. In cities like New York City, where police investigation, rape kit testing, and prosecution are highly proactive, 70 percent of rape cases result in arrests—triple the national average.[8]

DOCUMENTING THE USE OF PATIENT RESTRAINTS

Every day, approximately tens of thousands of hospitalized and long-term care patients in the United States are physically restrained. Many are injured from physical restraints, and some die as a direct result of their use. Because of these considerations, Congress and the Food and Drug Administration have enacted special rules governing the use of physical restraints.

Under interpretive guidelines established pursuant to the Nursing Home Reform Act in the Omnibus Reconciliation Act of 1987, healthcare organizations must justify the use of patient physical restraints in detailed patient care documentation. The FDA requires manufacturers of physical restraints to label them for use "by prescription only" in an attempt to minimize improper use of restraints.

Because of the inherent danger of misuse and neglect associated with physical restraints, providers must document the following prior to using patient restraints[9]:

- The use of restraints is clinically justified.
- Appropriate healthcare providers have been consulted and that less restrictive alternatives have been attempted and are inadequate.
- The patient's physical and mental conditions have been taken into account when deciding to use restraints. The restraints used are the least restrictive for the patient's protection, and that of relevant others.

Healthcare organization administrators and their supporting clinical and legal staff should develop protocols for the proper use of restraints. Appropriate justifications for the use of physical restraints might include the following:

- Combative patient behavior, posing a danger to the patient or others
- Patient elopement, where the patient's wandering has the potential to cause patient injury or injury to others
- Patient or surrogate request, with physician concurrence

Documentation considerations for using physical restraints include the following (consistent with federal and applicable state law):

- A physician must order the use of physical restraints, except in an emergency. In the absence of a physician on duty, a registered nurse can order their use temporarily, while he or she expeditiously seeks a verbal order from a physician.
- Verbal orders for physical restraints must be countersigned by the physician expeditiously (within 24 hours).
- The physician ordering physical restraints must document in the patient care record the patient's behavior justifying the use of restraints, the type of restraint to be used, the time period for its use, the frequency of checks on the patient, including the taking of the patient's vital signs, and conditions for removal of restraints.

Restraint orders must be reevaluated and rewritten at regular short intervals, which vary according to the patient care setting.

ELECTRONIC PATIENT CARE RECORDS (EHR)

In this age of rapid dissemination of information, more and more patient care information is being entered and stored electronically. President George W. Bush, in his January 2004 State of the Union address, promised to accelerate the development of electronic medical records (EMR) for everyone in the United States, a decade-long project that will cost $10 billion, but potentially save $170 billion (one-tenth of healthcare expenditures) annually. President Obama put President Bush's promises into action in February 2009 with the passage and implementation of the American Recovery and Reinvestment Act (ARRA), commonly known as the "stimulus package."[10]

The ARRA provides $19.5 billion in federal stimulus incentive funds over five years to encourage hospitals and medical doctors to convert more costly and cumbersome paper-based patient care record systems to electronic medical record systems. The maximum incentive available to each physician is $44,000, approximately equal to the average cost of converting a paper-based office system to an electronic medical records system. To participate in this federal incentive program, physicians must make "meaningful use" of electronic medical records, have at least 30 percent Medicare patients in their patient populations, and communicate diagnostic results with patients within 48 hours. Failure to convert to electronic medical records by 2014 carries a disincentive to hospitals and qualifying physicians—the loss of up to three percent of Medicare health services reimbursement.

There are a myriad of advantages to electronic health records for patients and for healthcare providers and organizations. For providers, the use of computers to record patient care data results in more legible and efficient documentation than in longhand. Most computer software programs offer templates that make electronic patient care documentation seemingly painless. Spelling and grammar check features and other error detection features minimize the likelihood of a mistake being made that could affect patient care.

Electronic medical records software can reveal if, on reevaluation, patients are making progress according to the initial plan of care. EMR software is commonly Medicare-specific, streamlining the electronic billing process for Medicare itself and for other third-party payer billing. It also can display graphic representations of patient outcomes for benchmarking to national quality standards and for research purposes.[11]

Tablet personal computers (PCs) and personal digital assistants (PDAs) ease electronic patient care documentation for mobile providers, such as those carrying out home-based patient care. Tablet PCs operate in Apple and Windows formats, and enable users to convert handwritten patient care notes into electronic print, using a digital pen.[12]

For patients, computerized patient care records offer many advantages over paper records. Patients may have to worry less about the loss of personal health information with electronic-format medical records. Patient health histories can be retrieved quickly by a provider linked to a patient database in a given healthcare facility. "Smart" (patient identification) cards, and even patient wristbands containing computerized memory chips, store complete patient health histories and care data. These data—available to healthcare professionals nationwide—make routine and emergency patient care more efficient and less costly.

There are potential disadvantages of computer-generated patient health records, too. Of primary concern is patient confidentiality. Access to patient databases must be limited to providers and others having an official need and right to know the information contained therein. Failure to safeguard patient information stored on computer—such as with a secure password access system—can lead to adverse administrative HIPAA action by the Office of Civil Rights, or civil tort liability for breach of patient confidentiality or intentional infliction of emotional distress associated with the unauthorized release of private patient information. Other disadvantages of electronic medical records include the fact that they may generate excessive patient information that may not be read by other healthcare providers compared to brief, handwritten notes, and eventually may alter the legal standard of care as they supplant paper-based patient care documentation as the "gold standard."[13]

Providers who use computers to create EMRs must be issued user names and passwords to perform their job functions. Users should select passwords that are difficult to steal—ones not related to a user's job or personal life. Users must not share their passwords with anyone—coworkers, supervisors, or even IT administrative personnel. Computer users and system managers are also urged to change passwords at regular intervals to prevent unauthorized access to patient care records.

With computerized patient record systems, there is also an increased danger that providers will be tempted to alter or erase prior patient entries, especially in the face of pending healthcare malpractice actions. Computer fraud experts can readily retrieve "lost" or erased files. Provider education about individual professional responsibility is the key to preventing spoliation of computerized patient care records. Risk managers should also consider installing system controls that do not permit alteration of original completed patient care record entries, only addendums in the form of new notation (i.e. the features in the Veterans Administration's Computerized Medical Records System, discussed below).

HIPAA's Security Rule, which took effect April 24, 2005, established new federal standards for security of PHI in electronic form: electronic medical records, email communications, and electronic claims transmissions, among other e-correspondence. Its 18 standards include required and optional specifications. No specific technologies are required to be implemented. Instead, each covered entity must first conduct a risk assessment of its operation, focusing on possible compromises to PHI security, then implement effective solutions to the challenges posed.[14]

The Veterans Administration's Computerized Medical Records System (CPRS) is a potential model for national standardized electronic medical records systems, offering onsite and remote users online access to patient health information, including sophisticated diagnostic imaging studies. CPRS and its VistA (Veterans Health Information Systems and Technology Architecture) platform won the prestigious 2006 Innovations in American Government Award.[15] (A demonstration model of the latest version of CPRS is at http://www.ehealth.va.gov/EHEALTH/CPRS_demo.asp.)

Photographic documentation of patient status and interventions is also being used increasingly. Surgeons, rehabilitation and wound care therapists, and others use photography to memorialize, among other findings, patient appearance before and after surgery, limb and spinal range of motion, postural alignment, and wound healing. Health record administrators must exercise special precautions to preserve photographic evidence until statutory record retention requirements are met. An additional consideration is the expense, manpower, and time involved in copying photographs for release to patients, their attorneys, insurers, and others.

Video documentation of patient status and interventions is also being used more frequently by healthcare professionals. A common example is the "day-in-the-life" videotape of a typical rehabilitation day for a tort plaintiff involved in litigation. In one medical malpractice case involving an allegation of negligent placement of a feeding catheter, *Georgacopoulos v. University of Chicago*, the court admitted a day-in-the-life videotape of the patient's "painful physical therapy session."[16] The court established a test for admission of this kind of videotape patient care documentation as follows:

1. The tape must depict an accurate representation of the patient's condition, circumstances, and rehabilitation.

2. The tape's value in the proceedings as relevant and probative evidence must outweigh any inflammatory effect that it might have on the jury.

3. The taped rehabilitation session must not amount to merely cumulative, or repetitive, evidence.

4. The depiction of the patient must be in good taste.

In *Georgacopoulos*, the court concluded that the videotape evidence of the patient–plaintiff's rehabilitation met the required tests and that the physical therapy session amounted to only a few minutes.

A serious consideration for health record administrators and risk managers is patient privacy. Videotaping of patient examination and/ or intervention in a facility requires explicit written informed consent, signed by the patient and/or the patient's legally appointed representative. Videotaped patient care documentation, like photographic, paper-based, and electronic format patient care documentation, must be retained in accordance with statutory, institutional, and customary requirements.

According to Dr. Steve Salvatore, MD, the primary health professional–computer relationship is the second most important health professional relationship (behind the health professional–patient relationship) in the 21st century.[17] Some patients are already storing their health records on the Internet, through companies such as PersonalMD.com, AboutMyHealth.net, and drkoop.com (founded by Dr. C. Everett Koop, former United States Surgeon General), among a growing number of others. A key advantage of such systems is ready access of patient historical information for healthcare providers, for both routine care and emergencies. A principal concern of patients and health professionals about such systems is the potential for a breach of patient privacy by third parties not having the right or a medical need for the information contained therein. Safeguards from encryption to PIN numbers for access to digital trails, indicating who has viewed patient records may help to limit or prevent invasions of privacy.[18]

HIPAA

The Health Insurance Portability and Accountability Act of 1996 (HIPAA)[19] is a federal law designed to ensure portability of employee health benefits when employees change jobs and a system for maximizing patient protected health information privacy.

HIPAA's provisions related to protected health information (PHI) privacy include the Privacy and Security Rules (discussed in this section) and the Electronic Data Transmission Standards (discussed under reimbursement later in this chapter).

The Privacy Rule, effective since April 14, 2003, is designed to prevent unauthorized and unwarranted disclosure of patient PHI. Healthcare systems, plans, providers, and clearinghouses that conduct financial transactions electronically must be committed to compliance with the letter and spirit of HIPAA in receiving, processing, storing, transmitting, and otherwise handling patient/client PHI.

HIPAA's privacy standards represent the first comprehensive federal guidelines for protection of PHI. Supplemental guidance and protections are found in state and local case law, statutes, and administrative rules and regulations. Protection extends to any individually identifiable health information, maintained or transmitted in any medium, held by any covered entity or business associate of a covered entity.

Covered entities must obtain adequate contractual assurances from business associates that the latter will appropriately safeguard patient PHI that comes to them. Examples of activities that may be conducted by business associates include benefit management, billing, claims processing, data analysis, quality improvement management, practice management, and utilization review. If a business associate is found to have violated HIPAA, the covered entity must first attempt to *cure* (correct) the *breach* (violation) of contract, and, if unsuccessful, terminate the contract with the noncompliant business associate and report the matter to the Secretary of the Department of Health and Human Services for follow-up administrative action.

Each employee, contractor, and consultant is a fiduciary, owing a personal duty to patients to take all reasonable steps pursuant to HIPAA to safeguard their PHI. All employees and other providers must receive HIPAA training during initial orientation and periodically thereafter to update their knowledge base about HIPAA.

Providers and entities covered by HIPAA must exercise reasonable caution under all circumstances to disclose only the minimum necessary amount of PHI to comply with their legal duties owed to patients and others.

On the first visit to any covered provider, all patients must be made aware of the facility's HIPAA Privacy Policy. Direct care providers must issue a Patient Notice of Privacy Practices to all patients at first contact, and make a good faith attempt to obtain patients' written acknowledgment of receipt of the document. In addition, providers must post their entire Patient Notice of Privacy Practices in their facility in a prominent location for patients to see. Exemplars of HIPAA Patient Notice of Privacy Practices documents in English and Spanish appear as **Exhibits 6–2** and **6–3**.

Exhibit 6–2 HIPAA Privacy Notification (Covered Entity, Workers' Compensation Practice)

ABC Rehabilitation Clinic
654 1st Avenue, SW
Majestic, USA 15551 (210) 555-HELP

CLINIC PRIVACY POLICY

Effective date: April 16, 2003

THIS NOTICE INFORMS YOU OF THE PROTECTIONS WE AFFORD TO YOUR PERSONAL HEALTH INFORMATION (PHI). PLEASE READ IT CAREFULLY.

Purpose: HIPAA, the Health Insurance Portability and Accountability Act of 1996, is a federal law addressing privacy and the protection of personal health information (PHI). This law gives you significant new rights as to how your PHI is used. HIPAA provides for penalties for misuse of PHI. As required by HIPAA, this notice explains how we are obliged to maintain the privacy of your PHI and how we are permitted, by law, to use and communicate it.

Maintenance of records: We utilize and communicate your PHI for the following reasons: treatment, reimbursement, and administrative medical operations.

- Treatment includes medical services delivered by professionals. Example: evaluation by a doctor or nurse.
- Reimbursement includes activities required for reimbursement for services, including, among other things, confirming insurance

coverage, sending bills and collection, and utilization review. Example: sending off a bill for services to your company for payment.

• Administrative medical operations include the business of managing the clinic, including, among other things, improving the quality of services, conducting audits, and client services. Example: patient satisfaction surveys.

We also are permitted to create and distribute anonymous medical information by removing all references to PHI.

All of the employees of this clinic may see your records, as needed. We use sign-in and sign-out logs, containing the names of our patients in the waiting room, and we telephone patients to confirm appointments. We place your folder in a plastic in-box (with your name hidden) in the hallway in front of your treatment room.

When making photocopies of your records, we have your folder in our sight at all times, until we file it away with other folders. The medical records area is limited to employees only. When we send your PHI by fax, we ensure to the maximum extent possible that the receiving fax is secure.

All other uses of your PHI require your written authorization, including sharing your PHI with family members or others. You have the right to revoke any authorization in writing, and we have the legal duty to comply with such a revocation, except to the extent that we have used your information in reliance on your previous authorization, or as required by law.

The right of patients to see, copy, and amend their medical records: To take advantage of these rights, please present your request in writing to the clinic Privacy Officer (see below). You have the right to see your medical records. We will try to give you access as quickly as possible, depending on our load. Within one week of your request, you may see your records in one of our offices, with the assistance of one of our employees. You have the right to make copies of your records. We have the right to charge for those copies. You may also petition the Privacy Officer for special limitations on the uses and communications of your PHI. We are not obliged to comply with such requests. If we agree, we have to comply with the request until you advise us in writing otherwise. You have the right to receive a copy of this notice, which we offer to you on your first visit. This notice, which is subject to change, is posted prominently in our waiting area.

Privacy Officer: The Privacy Officer for the clinic is _____ _____, RN. Please, speak with this employee about any question or complaint that you may have about your PHI. You may make special requests concerning your PHI.

Medical information shared with your employer: You have the right to a private consultation with your health professional. Healthcare records concerning illness or injury acquired on the job (worker's compensation) do not enjoy complete protection under privacy laws. Your employer has the right to know the details of your condition if it reflects on your ability to work. We will give the employer medical information pertinent to your work when it is authorized or necessary to comply with the worker's compensation legal system.

Correspondence with the patient: We will send correspondence to the address that you have given us, but you have the right to ask that we send correspondence to a different address.

Complaints: If you feel that your PHI has not been treated with privacy, you may communicate this concern to the clinic Privacy Officer. You also have the right to communicate any problem to the Secretary of Health and Human Services (of the federal government) without being worried about retaliation by this clinic. We ask that you first discuss the problem with our Privacy Officer. Thanks and welcome to ABC Clinic!

Exhibit 6–3 Privacy Notification, Workers' Compensation Setting (Spanish Version)

Clínica ABC de Rehabilitación
654 1st Avenue, SW
Majestic, USA 15551
(210) 555-HELP

NORMA DE PRIVACIDAD DE LA CLÍNICA

Effective date: April 16, 2003
ESTA NOTICIA LE INFORMA SOBRE LAS PROTECCIÓNES QUE TOMAMOS CON SU INFORMACIÓN MÉDICA.
HAZ FAVOR DE LEERLO CON CUIDADO.

Intento: HIPAA, el Health Insurance Portability and Accountability Act of 1996, es una ley federal que trata con la privacidad y protección de información personal médica (IPM). Está ley le da a usted, el paciente, derechos significantes nuevos sobre como se utiliza su IPM. HIPAA provee por penas por el mal uso de IPM. Como es requisito por HIPAA, esta norma explica como estamos obligado de mantener la privacidad de IPM y como estamos permitido usar y comunicar su IPM. Mantenamiento de los documentos: Utilizamos y comunicamos su IPM por las razones siguientes: el tratamiento, el pago, y las operaciones administrativas médicas.

- Tratamiento incluye servicios medicales entregados por profesionales. Ejemplo: evaluación por un médico o enfermera.
- Pago incluye actividades requisitas para el reembolso de servicios, incluyendo, entre otras cosas, confirmar los seguros, mandar facturas y colecionar, y análisis de utilización. Ejemplo: mandando una factura a su compañia de seguro para cobrar.
- Operaci—nes administrativas médicas que incluyen el negocio de administrar la clínica, el mejoramiento de la calidad de servicios, hacer auditorias, y servicio de clientes. Ejemplo: encuestas de satisfacción.

También podemos hacer y distribuir información médica anónima por quitar todas referencias a la IPM.

Todos los empleados de esta clínica pueden ver sus documentos, si necesitan verlos. Usamos planillas de firmar al entrar y salir, anunciamos los nombres de nuestros pacientes en la sala de espera, y llamamos a pacientes por teléfono para recordarles de sus citas. Pondremos su carpeta de documentos en un caja plástica (con nombre escondido) en el pasillo de su cuarto de tratamiento. Al hacer copias de sus documentos, tendremos la carpeta en nuestra vista hasta que lo guardamos con las otras carpetas. La area en que guardamos las carpetas está limitada a sólo los empleados.

Cuando mandamos sus documentos por fax, nos aseguramos lo más posible que el fax a donde lo mandamos está seguro. Todos otros usos de su IPM requiere su autorización escrito, incluyendo el compartamiento de su IPM con familiares u otras personas. Tiene el derecho de revocar su autorización en escrito, y tenemos la responsabilidad de cumplir con tal revocación, excepto al punto que ya hemos usado la información dependiente de su autorización anterior, o cuando tenemos que comunicar información por ley.

El derecho de los pacientes a ver, copiar y enmendar sus documentos mèdicos: Para ejecutar estos derechos, por favor presente su petición en escrito al Oficial de la Privacidad (vea abajo). Usted tiene el derecho de ver sus documentos médicos. Trataremos de rapidamente darle aceso, dependiente en lo ocupado que estemos. Entre una semana después de su solicitud, podrá ver los documentos en una sala de esta oficina, con la asistencia de un empleado. Tendrá el derecho de hacer copias. Tenemos el derecho de cobrar por las copias. También puede pedir al Oficial de la Privacidad peticiónes especiales sobre los usos y comunicaciónes de su IMP. No tenemos que cumplir con estas peticiónes. Si estamos de acuerdo, tenemos que seguir con la petición hasta que usted acuerde en escrito de quitarla. Tiene el derecho de tener una copia de esta noticia, que le ofrecemos en su primera visita a la clínica. Esta notica, que se puede cambiar, esta puesto prominentement en la sala de recepción.

Oficial de la Privacidad: El Oficial de la Privacidad de la clínica es _____ _____, RN. Por favor, hable con este empleado sobre cualquiera pregunta o queja que tenga sobre su IPM. Puede pedirle cosas en especial sobre su IPM.

Información médica compartida con su empleador: Usted tiene el derecho de tener una consulta privada con el médico. Los documentos de una enfermedad o herida adquirida en el trabajo (workers' comp) no están completamente protegidos por las leyes de la privacidad. Su empleador tiene el derecho de saber detalles de su condición si refleja su capacidad de trabajar. Le daremos información médica que pertenece al trabajo cuando es autorizado o necesario para cumplir con las leyes del sistema de indemnización laboral.

Correspondencia al paciente: Mandaremos cartas a la dirección que usted nos ha dado, pero tiene el derecho de pedir que las mandemos a otra dirección.

Quejas: Si usted piensa que su IPM no ha sido tratado con privacidad, usted puede comunicar este problema al Oficial de la Privacidad de la clínica. También tiene el derecho de comunicar cualquier problema al Secretario de Health and Human Services (en el gobierno federal) sin preocupaciónes de retaliación de esta clínica. Le rogamos que hables primeramente con el Oficial de la Privacidad. Gracias y bienvenido a la clínica ABC.

Normally, a covered entity (any provider filing reimbursement claims electronically) may use and disclose a patient's PHI for purposes of treatment, payment for services, and internal healthcare operations of the business, without the patient's authorization or consent. These disclosures are called *routine uses*. Regarding patient informed consent for routine uses of PHI, providers are required only to make a good faith effort to obtain patient/client informed consent for treatment, payment, and healthcare operations. Covered entities have wide discretion to design processes that mesh with their individual practices. Patients/clients have the right to request restrictions on the use or disclosure of their protected health information, but covered entities are not required to agree to such restrictions.

There are three general classifications of PHI disclosures under HIPAA. They are permissive and mandatory (both without patient authorization or consent), and authorized. Permissive disclosures include those necessary for treatment, payment, and operations (TPO). This includes, among other possibilities, communication between and among treatment team members, determination of coverage for health services, and peer/utilization review activities.

Required or mandatory disclosures are those made pursuant to legal mandates, such as a court order or state reporting statutes (for suspected abuse, communicable diseases [including sexually transmitted diseases], and gunshot wounds). Authorized disclosures encompass broad disclosure authority pursuant to valid written and signed patient authorization.

Regarding minors' PHI, the Privacy Rule generally allows a parent to have access to the medical records of his or her child, as his or her minor child's personal representative, when such access is not inconsistent with state or other laws. There are three situations when the parent would not be the minor's personal representative under the Privacy Rule. These exceptions are: (1) when the minor is the one who consents to care and the consent of the parent is not required under state or other applicable law, (e.g., when the minor is emancipated); (2) when the minor obtains care at the direction of a court or a person appointed by the court; and (3) when, and to the extent that, the parent agrees that the minor and the healthcare provider may have a confidential relationship. However, even in these exceptional situations, the parent may have access to the health record of the minor related to this treatment when state or other applicable law requires or permits such parental access.

The following are suggested standard operating procedures for clinics that are covered entities under HIPAA's Privacy Rule. This list is not intended to be comprehensive. In addition to appointing and adequately training a clinic Privacy Officer, all covered entities should brainstorm on a list of standard operating procedures to be implemented for their individual practices.

Suggested Standard Operating Procedures Pursuant to HIPAA's Privacy Rule

1. Staff will not allow patient records to be placed or to remain in open (public) view.

2. Staff will not discuss patient PHI within the hearing/perceptive range of third parties not involved in the patient's care.

3. Patients and other nonemployees/contractors/consultants are not permitted access to the patient records room.

4. Except where authorized, permitted, or required by law, PHI disclosures require HIPAA-compliant written patient/client authorizations and written requests by requestors for information.

5. Patient records may not be removed from the facility, except for transit to and from secure storage, or otherwise as authorized, permitted, or required by law.

6. Written requests by patients for their health records will be expeditiously honored.

7. Patient/client records may be placed in chart holders for clinic providers, provided that the following reasonable and appropriate measures are taken to protect the patient's privacy: limiting access to patient care areas and escorting nonemployees in the area, ensuring that the areas are supervised, and placing patient/client charts in chart holders with the front cover facing the wall rather than having protected health information about the patient visible to anyone who walks by.

8. Providers may leave phone messages for patients on their answering machines. Limit the amount of information disclosed

on the answering machine to clinic name and number, and any other information necessary to confirm an appointment, asking the individual to call back. It is permissible to leave a similar message with a family member or other person who answers the phone when the patient is not home.

9. The clinic is required to give the notice of its privacy policy to every individual receiving treatment no later than the date of first service delivery, and to make a good faith effort to obtain the individual's written acknowledgment of receipt of the notice.

10. The clinic is required to give the notice of its privacy policy to every individual receiving treatment no later than the date of its first service delivery, and to make a good faith effort to obtain the individual's written acknowledgment of receipt of the notice. The clinic also must post its entire privacy policy in the facility in a clear and prominent location where individuals are likely to see it, as well as make the notice available to those who ask for a copy. Copies of the clinic privacy notice are maintained in English and Spanish.

Providers covered by HIPAA may still utilize sign-in sheets for patients, and call out their names in waiting rooms, so long as PHI is not disclosed in these processes. Seeing someone in a waiting room and hearing one's name called constitute "incidental" disclosures that do not violate HIPAA, according to the Department of Health and Human Services. A sign-in sheet may not, however, list patients' diagnoses.

Providers may also transmit patient health records to other providers without patient authorization or consent, if the gaining providers are treating the patient for the same condition as the sending provider. This includes transfer of an entire patient health record (including documentation created by other providers), if reasonably necessary for treatment.

Providers are not normally required to document a "disclosure history" unless patient authorization is required for disclosure; however, it would be prudent risk management to create and maintain such a history. What is required is that covered providers and entities exercise reasonable caution under all circumstances to disclose only the minimum necessary amount of PHI in order to comply with their legal duties owed to patients and others.

The HIPAA Privacy Rule does not apply to entities that are workers' compensation insurers, administrative agencies, or employers, except to the extent they may otherwise be covered entities. These entities need access to the health information of individuals who are injured on the job or who have a work-related illness to process and adjudicate claims, and to coordinate care under workers' compensation systems. Generally, this health information is obtained from healthcare providers who are covered by the Privacy Rule.

The Privacy Rule recognizes the legitimate need of insurers and other entities involved in the workers' compensation systems to have access to individuals' health information as authorized by state or other laws. Because of the significant variability among such laws, the Privacy Rule permits disclosures of health information for workers' compensation purposes in the following number of different ways:

1. Disclosures Without Individual Authorization. The Privacy Rule permits covered entities to disclose protected health information to workers' compensation insurers, state administrators, employers, and other persons or entities involved in workers' compensation systems, without the individual's authorization under the following circumstances:

   a. As authorized by and to the extent necessary to comply with laws relating to workers' compensation or similar programs established by law that provide benefits for work-related injuries or illness without regard to fault. This includes programs established by the Black Lung Benefits Act, the Federal Employees' Compensation Act, the Longshore and Harbor Workers' Compensation Act, and the Energy Employees' Occupational Illness Compensation Program Act. See 45 CFR 164.512(*l*).

   b. To the extent the disclosure is required by State or other law. The disclosure must comply with and be limited to what the law requires. See 45 CFR 164.512(a).

   c. For purposes of obtaining payment for any health care provided to the injured or ill worker. See 45 CFR 164.502(a)(1)(ii) and the definition of "payment" at 45 CFR 164.501.

2. Disclosures With Individual Authorization. In addition, covered entities may disclose protected health information to workers' compensation insurers and others involved in workers' compensation systems where the individual has provided his or her authorization for the release of the information to the entity. The authorization must contain the elements and otherwise meet the requirements specified at 45 CFR 164.508.

3. Minimum Necessary. Consistent with HIPAA's Privacy Rule main theme, covered entities are required reasonably to limit the amount of protected health information disclosed under 45 CFR 164.512(*l*) to the minimum necessary to accomplish the workers' compensation purpose. Under this requirement, protected health information may be shared for such purposes to the full extent authorized by State or other law. In addition, covered entities are required reasonably to limit the amount of protected health information disclosed for payment purposes to the minimum necessary. Covered entities are permitted to disclose the amount and types of protected health information that are necessary to obtain payment for health care provided to an injured or ill worker. Where a covered entity routinely makes disclosures for workers' compensation purposes under 45 CFR 164.512(*l*) or for payment purposes, the covered entity may develop standard protocols as part of its minimum necessary policies and procedures that address the type and amount of protected health information to be disclosed for such purposes. Where protected health information is requested by a state workers' compensation or other public official, covered entities are permitted to reasonably rely on the official's representations that the information requested is the minimum necessary for the intended purpose. See 45 CFR 164.514(d)(3)(iii)(A). Covered entities are not required to make a minimum necessary determination when disclosing protected health information as required by state or other law, or pursuant to the individual's authorization. See 45 CFR 164.502(b).

HIPAA-related patient complaints should first be directed to an organization's HIPAA Privacy Officer. A complaint may also be filed with the Office of Civil Rights, U.S. Department of Health and Human Services (DHHS).

DHHS requires the following in a written complaint:

1. Complainant's full name and residential and email addresses, home and work phone numbers

2. Name, address, and phone number of entity violating complainant's PHI

3. Description of the PHI violation

4. Complainant's signature and date

5. Necessary reasonable accommodations, as applicable

An alleged PHI violator is prohibited from taking retaliatory action against a complainant. Potential sanctions for HIPAA Privacy Rule violations include civil and criminal penalties. Civil penalties of between $100 and $25,000 per violation are enforced by the Office of Civil Rights, Department of Health and Human Services. Criminal sanctions of 1 to 10 years imprisonment and $50,000 to $250,000 fines are enforced by the Department of Justice.

LEGAL ISSUES ASSOCIATED WITH REIMBURSEMENT DOCUMENTATION

Effective documentation is crucial for reimbursement for healthcare service delivery by third-party payers. In the implied contract between a healthcare provider and a patient, the implicit promise of the patient is to pay the reasonable cost of services rendered. (In return, the healthcare professional promises to use his or her best clinical judgment and skills to effect an optimal therapeutic result.)

There are three potential sources for payment for healthcare services. First-party payment equates to self-payment by the patient. Second-party payment implies that a healthcare provider absorbs the cost of care him or herself, as in *pro bono* (no charge) care rendered to indigent patients. Third-party reimbursement is payment for health services by insurers, including Medicare, Medicaid, and TriCare—the principal federal public third-party payers.

The concept of health insurance centers on the legal premise that the enormous expense of healthcare delivery—especially for catastrophic injuries or illnesses—should be diluted through risk pooling among thousands or millions of subscribers. In this way, a pool of group funds (including reserves) is available to meet such challenges.

Medicare[20] is the largest third-party payer for health services. In existence only since 1966, Medicare spending in 2009 exceeded $425.5 billion, a 7.5-fold increase from 25 years ago, when, in 1983, Medicare's budget was $52.6 billion.[21]

Part A Medicare, funded by the Hospital Insurance Trust, pays for inpatient hospital care, care in skilled nursing facilities, home health services, and hospice care. Part A coverage is universal for Medicare beneficiaries. Part B optional coverage pays for outpatient physician and nonphysician services, and requires monthly premium payments ($110.50 in 2010).

Medicare covered beneficiaries include those persons age 65 years or older, 100 percent disabled for at least 24 months, or having amyotrophic lateral sclerosis (i.e., Lou Gehrig's disease) or end-stage renal disease requiring dialysis and possible transplant.

Like hospitals for inpatient services, skilled nursing facilities (SNFs) and home health agencies (HHAs) are under prospective (lump-sum) payment for services. Home health service providers utilize OASIS-C, the Outcome and Assessment Information Set, as part of initial adult home-bound patient care documentation. OASIS-C items describe patient health status and function. HHAs must utilize this lengthy database as a condition of participation in Medicare and Medicaid. Medicare's Web site (http://www.Medicare.gov) describes OASIS-C in detail and offers a list of Medicare-certified home health agencies for each region of the country.

As part of cost containment, the Balanced Budget Act of 1997 imposed outpatient rehabilitation therapy caps on physical (shared with speech therapy) and occupational therapy of $1,590 per year per patient. That reimbursement cap was alternately enforced or suspended through 2010, when Congress enacted an across-the-board 30-plus-percent reduction in reimbursement for outpatient therapy services reimbursement, placing the cap at $1,811 for 2011.[22]

In any clinical practice setting, documentation for reimbursement requires price *coding*. Coding serves the several following functions:

1. It is a language based on guidelines.

2. It is directly tied to patient care documentation.

3. It is a method by which reimbursement for services ensues.

4. It serves as a description of health professional services rendered to patients.

There are financial, legal, and ethical considerations to coding health-care services. Proper coding facilitates prompt reimbursement for patient care. Inappropriate coding may lead to civil and criminal liability for fraud. It is unethical to intentionally miscode services.

Coding may be based on any one, or a combination of inputs from the following systems. ICD-9, the *International Classification of Diseases*, ninth edition, includes numeric and alphanumeric codes for numerous patient diagnoses. CPT-4, *Current Procedural Terminology*, fourth edition, a proprietary system of the American Medical Association, includes five-character numeric codes assigned to virtually every healthcare service.

For rehabilitation professionals, CPT codes are mostly found in the 97000 (Physical Medicine and Rehabilitation) section. There are timed (15 minute-average, 8-minute minimum intervals) and untimed codes. Untimed codes include the range of therapeutic activities from the complex (patient evaluation) to the mundane (hot/cold pack application). Some passive treatments, such as hot pack application, are not normally reimbursed by third-party payers as a matter of cost-containment policy.

Coded procedures are valued based on the resources required to perform each procedure. Valuation inputs include complexity of the procedure and work effort expended and practice expenses and costs like overhead and professional liability insurance. CMS uses the Resource-Based Relative Value System (RBRVS) for assessing the value of Medicare outpatient medical services.

Patient care documentation substantiates the medical necessity for rehabilitative professional services. Providers must clearly delineate the need for skilled rehab services and demonstrate that such services are provided each time a patient is seen. Documentation must also demonstrate progress toward achievement of functional goals delineated in initial and reevaluations, and a patient's response to interventions. The reasonableness of time, frequency, and duration of interventions must also be well documented in order to be reimbursed for care. Regular (at least weekly) progress notes supplement daily care notes. Such notation must be clearly written and signed and dated by a licensed rehabilitation professional or legal designee.

The Final Rule for the HIPAA Electronic Transactions and Code Set Standards was published February 20, 2003. The rule requires covered entities to use a standardized HIPAA-compliant format (either CPT or HCPCS codes, not ICD-9 procedure codes) for electronic billing.

One important legal issue in healthcare reimbursement is whether a demand for third-party reimbursement by a healthcare provider and/or organization constitutes larceny, or theft, by fraud or deception. *Fraud* is defined as a false misrepresentation of a material fact, made with the intent to deceive, which causes another person to take some action detrimental to his or her own (or the public's) interest. A fraudulent misrepresentation can be the basis for administrative, civil, or criminal legal action against the person committing fraud. *Larceny by fraud* involves theft of money, goods, services, or property by deception.

Elements of fraud:

   1. A misrepresentation of fact

   2. Made with an intent to deceive

On which another person relies to his or her (or the public's) legal detriment
Larceny by fraud:
Theft of money, goods, services, or property by deception

According to the National Health Care Anti-Fraud Association, healthcare reimbursement fraud accounts for up to $100 billion of the annual $450 billion in Medicare healthcare expenditures in the United States.[23] The Office of the Inspector General of the federal Department of Health and Human Services (DHHS), as well as complementary state agencies, have recently accelerated investigation and prosecution of healthcare reimbursement fraud by providers and organizations. In 2010, the Department of Justice launched the Web site StopMedicareFraud.gov, which encourages patients, providers and others to report Medicare fraud by healthcare providers and organizations to federal authorities for prosecution.

Healthcare providers and organizations commit fraud against Medicare, Medicaid, TriCare, commercial third-party payers, workers' compensation agencies, and other entities, through their billing practices. Billing practices that can result in an allegation of fraud include knowingly filing false claims for reimbursement.

Practices that might constitute reimbursement fraud include the following:

1. Filing claims for health professional services not actually rendered, such as for patient "no shows," called *phantom billing*

2. Violations of "antikickback" and self-referral statutes

3. Overutilization (*unbundling*) of healthcare-related products and services paid for by third-party payers

4. *Upcoding* (miscategorizing) procedural terminology codes to enhance reimbursement

5. Failing to code two or more rehabilitation patients receiving 1:1 direct skilled care simultaneously under the less lucrative group therapy code (97150)

Inadequate patient care documentation may give rise to, and support an allegation of, third-party reimbursement fraud, leading to liability or settlement of charges with the federal Department of Health and Human Services. Penalties for a finding of reimbursement fraud can range from civil fines and liability; criminal convictions, including the imposition of criminal monetary fines; administrative penalties, including exclusion from participation in Medicare, Medicaid, or other federal and private third-party payer systems, and adverse licensing and/or certification action by federal, state, and private agencies; and professional association adverse actions for ethical violations.

MANDATORY REPORTING REQUIREMENTS

Healthcare providers engaged in primary care delivery are required by every state to report certain findings or good faith suspicions to state or federal authorities, including evidence of child, spouse, or elderly abuse; certain communicable diseases; and defective medical devices. Providers who carry out primary care—especially nonphysician providers, who may not be aware of their reporting obligations—should consult legal counsel to obtain a current summary of their state law on mandatory reporting requirements.

Abuse

Healthcare professionals have been sued both for the failure to report suspected or actual abuse and for the act of reporting suspected or actual abuse. Some state statutes provide absolute immunity for providers who report abuse found incident to their official healthcare duties, whereas others offer only a qualified immunity, based on a showing of good faith. A few states have no statutory universal abuse reporting requirements, or make such reporting voluntary.

Documentation of findings supporting a conclusion of abuse must be carefully and objectively spelled out in the patient care record. Documentation of the actual reporting of abuse, however, may be more appropriately memorialized in an office memorandum or in some file other than the patient care record, consistent with state or federal legal requirements. Remember that statements that are made by the patient for the purpose of diagnosis and/or intervention or that constitute extemporaneous "excited utterances" should be carefully transcribed verbatim into the patient care record to protect the patient's health and legal interests, because these statements may constitute admissible *hearsay* evidence against a perpetrator in a subsequent civil or criminal legal action.

Providers must be educated about the physical and psychological signs of abuse, including: unexplained injuries, malnutrition, withdrawal, and poor socialization. And they must not breach their fiduciary duty owed to patients under their care by failing to report abuse when they see or suspect it.

Occupational and Communicable Injury and Diseases

The timely detection, treatment, and monitoring of occupational diseases (e.g., asbestosis, carpal tunnel syndrome, and lead poisoning) and infectious diseases (including tuberculosis and venereal diseases) is crucial to the maintenance of individual and public health and safety. State legislatures, pursuant to their constitutional "police power" to protect public health, safety, and welfare, mandate that certain occupational and infectious diseases be reported by healthcare providers (and other professionals) to designated public health agencies at the local or state level. These reporting requirements are permissible exceptions to the duty of confidentiality owed by healthcare professionals to patients.

As with child, spouse, and elderly abuse, primary healthcare providers are legally responsible for complying with mandatory injury and disease reporting requirements. As the adage goes, "Ignorance of the law is no excuse for noncompliance." Since 1992, the Occupational Safety and Health Administration (OSHA) has required health professional employers to maintain records of employee exposure to blood-borne pathogens for the duration of the exposee's employment plus 30 years.[24] Providers must consult with their legal advisors for up-to-date statutory reporting requirements in their individual states.

Defective Medical Devices

Under the Safe Medical Devices Act of 1990, which became effective on November 28, 1991, healthcare facilities must report to the FDA and/or equipment manufacturers any cases involving patient injury in which there is a "reasonable suggestion" that a piece of medical equipment contributed to the death or serious injury of the patient.[25] Under this law, a healthcare organization must designate a person to write such a report (probably the risk manager or safety committee chairperson), which must be submitted within 10 working days of an adverse patient incident involving medical equipment. The report is forwarded directly to the FDA for death cases (as well as to the equipment manufacturer) and to the equipment manufacturer for serious injury cases (or to the FDA, if the identity of the manufacturer is unknown).

These reports enjoy qualified (limited) federal statutory immunity from use in civil litigation. This immunity probably was mandated to encourage the reporting of possibly faulty medical devices to federal authorities, so that warnings can be promptly issued to save lives.

PATIENT DISCHARGE DOCUMENTATION

Discharge planning for hospitalized patients is a multidisciplinary, coordinated process that requires careful documentation. Hospital patients often require follow-up skilled nursing facility, rehab hospital, outpatient or home care, and the coordination of these interventions should be noted in discharge nursing, physical and occupational therapy, social service, physician, and other relevant inpatient care documentation. In addition to serving to optimize quality patient care, proper notation of discharge instructions and coordinated follow-up care may serve as important evidence of quality and quantity of care rendered, in the event of an ensuing legal healthcare malpractice action alleging abandonment or other forms of professional negligence.

If home exercise or other interventions are to be used by a patient after discharge from immediate care, then written, personalized handouts should be issued to the patient. The fact that such materials have been issued to the patient and a summary of the teaching imparted to the patient and/or family/significant others should be documented in the patient's discharge note by the appropriate service.

If clinical information about a patient is to be sent to outside agencies or providers to facilitate home or outpatient care, then the patient's consent to release pertinent records should be secured before the patient is discharged. Patient follow-up appointments for reexamination and follow-up care also must be well documented, and the patient given appropriate appointment slips.

For discharged outpatients seen in clinics such as physical or occupational therapy pursuant to physician referral, the therapist responsible for the patient's care should forward a discharge summary to the referring physician on discharge. An example of such a letter appears as **Exhibit 6–4**.

Exhibit 6–4 Example of an Outpatient Discharge Report

Physical Therapy Services
ABC Rehabilitation Center
New Wave, California

Date: _____

(Referring Physician's Address)
Subject: Discharge Report
Patient Name: _____
Dear Dr. _____:

This letter is a discharge report on your patient, _____,
referred on _____ for the following outpatient physical therapy services: _____.

- Course and Duration of Treatment: _____
- Summary of Discharge Evaluation: _____
- Home Care Instructions/Needs: _____
- Follow-up Re-evaluation Instructions: _____
- Additional Comments: _____

Thank you for referring this interesting and pleasant patient to us for care.

Sincerely,
Reggie Hausenfus, PT Chief Physical Therapist

PATIENT NONCOMPLIANCE, DISENGAGEMENT, AND ABANDONMENT

As part of the implied contract of care between patient and provider, healthcare clinicians should explain the importance of compliance with instructions to patients during the initial visit and document what is said to the patient and the patient's responses. Providers should have in effect a written policy regarding patient responsibility for compliance with interventions. Providers should also consider including tactful reminders about attendance and compliance policies on patient appointment slips.

Every facility should have a written policy in effect regarding termination of the patient–provider relationship. Failure to comply with interventions and instructions may be a justification for disengaging from care for a patient. Although a provider has almost unlimited discretion to elect whether to form a professional relationship with a patient, the provider must comply with certain legal rules to terminate an existing health professional–patient relationship properly.

Termination of the provider–patient relationship is justified when the patient makes a knowing, voluntary election to end the relationship, either unilaterally or jointly with the provider. A provider may unilaterally choose to end the professional relationship with the patient when a cure has resulted from intervention, or when the patient, in the clinician's professional judgment, has achieved maximal benefit from intervention. This latter situation requires careful documentation in the patient care record that will withstand legal scrutiny in the event of a healthcare malpractice action. Also, whenever a clinician has provided patient care pursuant to a physician referral, the clinician should communicate in writing to the referring entity that the patient has been discharged.

Patient noncompliance, and even a personality conflict between provider and patient, can form appropriate reasons to discharge or transfer a patient. Under these circumstances, the provider must do the following:

1. Give advance notice to the patient (and the referring entity, if any) of the provider's intent to disengage from care.

2. If continuing care is needed, give the patient a reasonable time before terminating the professional relationship to find a suitable new provider. (A prudent risk management measure would be to assist the patient in finding a suitable substitute provider and document in an office memorandum the steps taken to assist the patient.)

3. On discharge, carefully draft and send to the patient a disengagement letter, coordinated through your facility or personal legal advisor. This type of letter may prevent the healthcare malpractice statute of limitations from being *tolled*, or suspended, because of a patient claim of "continuing care."

4. Carefully document in the patient care record the patient's status at the time of discharge.

5. Expeditiously transfer copies of the patient's records (but not any risk management-focused office memoranda or any incident reports involving the patient) to the follow-on provider and offer to communicate with the new provider telephonically about pertinent clinical information, consistent with written consent by the patient pursuant to HIPAA.

WITHDRAWAL OF LIFE SUPPORT/DNR GUIDELINES

The withholding or withdrawal of life-sustaining treatment and support and do-not-resuscitate (DNR) orders are distinct clinical considerations that need to be addressed separately. Both judgments now largely fall within the administrative ambit of the Patient Self-Determination Act, which has already been introduced in this chapter. Some situations, however, fall outside of the jurisdiction of that statute, requiring consideration by providers of other complex statutes, regulations, and common law court precedent. This brief overview of DNR orders is intended only to be a limited introduction to a complicated area of healthcare law and professional ethics.

A DNR order precludes the otherwise automatic initiation of cardiopulmonary resuscitative efforts for a patient. The order does not affect the provision of any other substantive care such as life support and other treatment decisions.

A DNR order may be appropriate in one of two situations: to respect the free choice of a patient with full mental and legal capacity or the valid decision of a surrogate decision maker, or when, in the judgment of the attending physician, resuscitative efforts would be futile.[26–28] An order to withhold or withdraw life-sustaining therapeutic interventions may be appropriate for patients who are either terminal or in a persistent "vegetative state."

In either case, careful documentation of specific orders by the attending physician is required, as well as careful documentation in the patient's progress notes of the following:

- The rationale or justification for such a decision
- A brief description of the patient's physical condition and mental/ legal capacity to make an advance directive decision
- Any discussion about the order with the patient and/or the patient's family and surrogate decision maker, if they are not one and the same
- Any input from an institutional ethics committee and/or ethics consultants

Physicians, consultants, and supportive providers may have to rely on what is documented in a patient's treatment record about DNR or life-support decisions in defending a wrongful death legal action. In respect of patient autonomy and for the legal protection of providers, this documentation must be accurate and comprehensive.

TELEHEALTH DOCUMENTATION ISSUES

Telehealth involves computerized information transfer systems and technology used to transmit patient care and related data to distant providers having an imminent need for the information conveyed. It poses great promise and potential problems for patients and healthcare providers and organizations. For patients, providers, and healthcare organizations, the rapid dissemination of vital patient care or educational or research information to providers may result in more efficacious patient care outcomes that are both more convenient and at lower cost.

Transmission of patient care information via the Internet or similar media carries the same risks of breach of confidentiality as does transmission of any other information through these media, except that the nature of the information potentially compromised is highly personal and sensitive. Adequate steps, including the prominent display of privacy warnings within such transmissions, must be undertaken by healthcare providers and organizations to meet fiduciary duties owed to patients under their care. Whether telehealth or *distance healthcare delivery* will provide the same (or better) quality of professional service delivery and satisfaction to patients is an open question, whose answer remains to be developed and seen.

For licensed primary healthcare professionals, the issue of unlicensed practice in states in which providers are not licensed accompanies interstate telehealth consultation and practice. Penalties for a finding of unlicensed healthcare practice may include administrative, civil, criminal, and professional association adverse actions. Ways to comply with local licensure requirements include licensure by endorsement, special registration, among others.[29] Currently, there is available limited reimbursement for telehealth consultations by providers in rural health professional shortage areas (HPSAs).

More and more, pharmaceuticals are being offered for sale to patients over the Internet.[30] Such practice, while convenient, may violate state licensure and federal prescription laws. In addition, because as many as one-tenth of patient admissions to hospitals involve adverse drug reactions,[31] Internet pharmacies may face liability for health professional negligence (including patient abandonment) for failing to be available to monitor their customers and to offer advice in drug-related emergencies.

CHAPTER SUMMARY

Healthcare providers—particularly those primary physician and nonphysician providers examining and intervening on behalf of patients in clinical practice—face complex healthcare legal issues on a daily basis. HIPAA compliance is required of all healthcare entities that bill electronically for services. Its rules are complex and require constant monitoring for ongoing compliance. Administrative compliance with HIPAA may add 10 percent or more to the total time allotted for patient care. Healthcare organization and system administrators and risk managers should ensure that these clinicians and their support staffs receive ongoing legal instruction on their formidable responsibilities in areas such as patient advance directives, documenting and reporting adverse incidents, documenting the treatment of sexual assault and otherwise abused patients, compliance with mandatory reporting requirements, discharge and disengagement documentation, and ethical and legal considerations surrounding DNR/withdrawal of life support orders, among a myriad of other considerations.

NOTES AND REFERENCES

1. The Patient Self-Determination Act, 42 U.S.C. Section 1395cc(f).

2. A *living will* is a legal document, signed by a patient, that states the patient's desires regarding life-sustaining measures to be taken in the event that the patient becomes mentally and legally incapacitated. Living will statutes are in effect in all states. Most states require a patient to be both mentally and legally incapacitated and terminal for a living will to become operative. Some states allow a living will to become activated when a patient is in a "persistent vegetative state."

3. *A durable power of attorney for healthcare decision-making* is a legal document, signed by a patient, that delegates healthcare decision-making to an agent of the patient's choice in the event that the patient becomes mentally and legally incapacitated. The patient executing a durable power of attorney normally may designate anyone—a spouse, relative, or friend—as his or her healthcare decision-maker.

4. *An out-of-hospital do-not-resuscitate order* is a state-approved document executed by a competent person with a terminal medical

condition. It is intended to prevent unwanted resuscitative measures by others away from a medical treatment facility.

5. *A declaration for mental health treatment* is a declaratory document executed by a competent person concerning future mental health treatment options for that person. Depending on state law, two witnesses who will not benefit from the declarant's will must also sign the document.

6. Larsen EJ, Eaton TA. The limits of advance directives: A history and assessment of the Patient Self-Determination Act. *Wake Forest Law Review.* 1997; 32(2):249–293.

7. See, e.g., Federal Rules of Evidence 803(2) and 803(4), which reads: The following (is) not excluded by the hearsay rule, even though the declarant is available as a witness: (2) Excited utterance. A statement relating to a startling event or condition made while the declarant was under the stress of excitement caused by the event or condition. . . . (4) Statements for purposes of medical diagnosis or treatment. Statements made for purposes of medical diagnosis or treatment and describing medical history, or past or present symptoms, pain, or sensations, or the inception or general character of the cause or external source thereof insofar as reasonably pertinent to diagnosis or treatment.

8. Keteyian A. Rape in America: Justice Defined. Nov. 9, 2009. CBS News, New York. Accessed July 3, 2011, from http://www.cbsnews .com/stories/2009/11/09/cbsnews_investigates/main5590118 .shtml

9. Clinical Issues: Patient Restraints. Washington State Department of Health. Nov. 12, 2010 (search title on homepage). Accessed July 3, 2011, from http://www.doh.wa.gov

10. American Reinvestment and Recovery Act of 2009. 8 United States Code Section 1101 *et seq.*

11. On the Record. *Facets.* Pittsburgh, PA: University of Pittsburgh Press; 2004:20–22.

12. McCormack J. Practices embrace tablet PCs. *Humana's Your Practice.* 2004:19–20.

13. Kern SI. Hidden Malpractice Dangers in EMRs. *Medscape.* May 4, 2009:1–3. Accessed July 4, 2011, from http://www.ctimedsys.com/HiddenMalpractice.pdf

14. Security Standards for the Protection of Electronic Protected Health Information ("Security Rule"). *Federal Register* 2003; 68(34): 8334–8381. Accessed July 4, 2011, from http://aspe.hhs.gov/admnsimp/final/fr03-8334.pdf

15. See United States Department of Veterans Affairs. VistA monograph. Accessed July 4, 2011, from http://www.informatics-review.com/wiki/index.php/Veterans_Health_Information_Systems_and_Technology_Architecture_(VistA). Accessed June 20, 2010.

16. *Georgacopoulos v. University of Chicago*, 504 N.E.2d 830 (111. App. Ct. 1987), at 832.

17. CNN Headline News, August 14, 1999.

18. Chase M. Patients' next choice: where to keep files stored on the Internet. *Wall Street Journal.* August 16, 1999:B1.

19. Health Insurance Portability and Accountability Act of 1996, Public Law 104-191, 45 Code of Federal Regulations, Part 160, Subparts A, E, Part 164.

20. Title XVIII, Social Security Act of 1965, 42 United States Code Sections 1395 *et seq.*

21. Health and Human Services. HHS proposes a $891,597,000 budget for fiscal year 2012. Accessed August 14, 2011, from http://www.hhs.gov/about/FY2012budget/fy2012bib.pdf

22. Medicare Makes Deeper Cuts to Rehabilitation Services. American Physical Therapy Association, Alexandria, VA; Nov. 2, 2010.

23. National Health Care Anti-Fraud Association. Accessed July 4, 2011, from http://www.nhcaa.org

24. *Code of Federal Regulations*, Section 1910.1030, 1996.

25. The Safe Medical Devices Act of 1990, 21 United States Code Sections 301note, 321, 360d, and 360hh *et seq.*

26. Guidelines for the appropriate use of do-not-resuscitate orders. Council on Ethical and Judicial Affairs, American Medical Association. *JAMA.* 1991; 265:1868–1871.

27. Biegler P. Should patient consent be required to write a do-not-resuscitate order? *Journal of Medical Ethics.* 2003; 29:359–363.

28. Becker G, Blum H. Medical futility: the doctor caught between the demands for and the limitations of treatment. *Deutsche Med Wochenschr.* 2004; 129:1694–1697.

29. Goldberg, AS. Taking healthcare to the patient–telemedicine delivers. *Health Law Digest.* 1999; 27:3–10.

30. Martin TW. More doctors are prescribing medicines online. *Wall Street Journal.* April 20, 2010:D2.

31. Fischman J. Drug bazaar: getting medicine off the Web is easy, but dangerous. *U.S. News and World Report,* June 21, 1999; 58–62.

ADDITIONAL SUGGESTED READINGS

American Health Information Management Association. Accessed July 4, 2011, from http://www.ahima.org/

Berry G. Keeping records secure. *Advance for Physical Therapists.* 1998:13.

Brimer M. Making the move to electronic documentation. *PT: Magazine of Physical Therapy.* 1998; 6:58–62.

Buppert C. Electronic Medical Records: 18 Ways to Reduce Legal Risks. *Medscape,* January 13, 2010. Accessed July 4, 2011, from http://www.medscape.com/viewarticle/714812

Conrad, DA. Lessons to apply to national comprehensive healthcare reform. *American Journal of Managed Care.* 2009; 15:S306–S312.

Cowan AE, Katz HS. HIPAA and the practice of law. *Texas Bar Journal.* 2004: 962–963.

Dombi WA. The new age of opportunity and risk: Medicare PPS. *Caring.* 2001; 20(3):6–8.

Erwin J. Keeping track: patient wristbands hold medical records. *Healthweek.* August 17, 1998:8.

Ferrarini EM. HIPAA tips. Advance for Physical Therapy & Rehab Medicine. Accessed July 4, 2011, from http://physical-therapy.advanceweb.com/Article/HIPAA-Tips-5.aspx

Hillestad R, Bigelow J, Bower A, Girosis F, Melili R, Scoville R. Can electronic medical record systems transform health care? *Health Affairs*. 2005; 24(5):1103–1117.

Jha AK, DesRoches CM, Campbell EG, et al. Use of electronic health records in U.S. hospitals. *N Engl J Med*. 2009; 360:1628–1638.

Lipton-Dibner W. Getting Doctors and Staff On Board With EHR.. *Medscape*. Sept. 2, 2009. Accessed July 4, 2011, from http://www.pro-impact.com/pdfs/Doctors-staff-EHR.pdf

Ramsaroop SD, Reid MC, Adelman MD. Completing an advance directive in the primary care setting: what do we need for success? *Journal of the American Geriatrics Society*. 2007; 55(2):277–283.

Scott RW. Incident reports: protecting the record. *PT: Magazine of Physical Therapy*. 1998; 4:24–25.

Scott RW. *Medical Spanish: A New Approach*. Sudbury, MA: Jones and Bartlett Publishers; 2008.

Sullivan GH. The right way to fill out an incident report. *RN*. 1988; 51:53–55.

Tidd CW. A process of putting the PPS patient first. *Caring*. 2001; 20(3):10–13.

United States Department of Health and Human Services. How to File a Complaint. Accessed July 4, 2011, from http://www.hhs.gov/ocr/privacy/hipaa/complaints/index.html

United States Department of Health and Human Services. Understanding Health Information Privacy. Accessed July 4, 2011, from http://www.hhs.gov/ocr/privacy/hipaa/understanding/

United States Department of Health and Human Services, Agency for Healthcare Research and Quality. Homepage. Accessed July 4, 2011, from http://www.ahrq.gov.

Vandagriff DP. Securing your data. *ABA Journal*. 1994; 80:58–59.

Wasserman R. Still hip to HIPAA? Advance for Physical Therapy & Rehab Medicine. 2004; 15(24):29–30. Accessed July 4, 2011, from http://physical-therapy.advanceweb.com/Article/Still-Hip-to-HIPAA.aspx

Weiler J. State-of-the-art home care documentation. *Advance for Physical Therapy & Rehab Medicine*. 1998:8–10, 26. Accessed July 4, 2011, from http://physical-therapy.advanceweb.com/Article/State-of-the-Art-Home-Care-Documentation.aspx

What's happening with HIPAA? *Texas Medicine Records*. 2003; 99:19–20.

REVIEW CASE STUDIES

1. X, an outpatient with a diagnosis of left shoulder adhesive capsulitis, arrives at the physical therapy clinic, XYZ Hospital, for his third treatment of "moist heat, followed by passive mobilization and active assistive exercises, followed by ice pack p.r.n." Before applying the heat, the physical therapist assistant, Y, notices a

2-in.-diameter blister at patient X's right acromioclavicular joint and inquires about it. Patient X states that Y had left the heat pack on his shoulder too long during his last treatment 2 days ago, and as a result, he sustained the burn. What does Y do?

2. It is December 26, 201x. C, an 89-year-old patient, presents to the emergency department of ABC Hospital, Lake Frio, Michigan, for examination and treatment for what her daughter-in-law, D, reports to have been a fall down three stairs onto her outstretched hands this morning. Patient C is reticent when questioned about the fall; however, D volunteers that patient C is frequently disposed to fall and bruise herself. Patient C's symptoms include emaciation, bruising and scratches over the dorsum of her hands and forearms, and painful bilateral shoulder active-assistive range of motion. Patient C is dressed in a sleeveless cotton dress. As emergency department head nurse, what advice would you offer to the intern evaluating patient C for treatment?

DISCUSSION: REVIEW CASE STUDIES

1. Y should withhold application of the heat treatment and immediately notify her supervising physical therapist about the incident. Heat pack burns account for a significant proportion of claims and lawsuits against physical therapists. Because Y observed patient X's condition and heard patient X's statements about attribution of cause, Y should write the incident report. In it, she should carefully document what she saw and heard. An appropriate entry describing the occurrence might be:

> Patient X arrived for treatment of moist heat and exercise at 1415 hours, Sept. 19, 201x. After patient X removed his shirt, I noticed a 1 7/8-in.-diameter round blister at his right acromioclavicular joint. The blister's periphery was surrounded with erythema. The wound was dry. Patient X stated to me, "You left the heat pack on too long during my last treatment, and I got burned." I notified Mary Therapist, P.T., who examined patient X and ordered his treatment withheld for now. Mary Therapist consulted with Dr. S

in the Acute Care Clinic, who agreed to examine patient X this afternoon. Follow-up pending.

Y was correct not to speculate as to the cause of patient X's burn or to admit fault and apologize for it in the incident report. Y's supervisor or the risk manager will determine cause during an investigation, and Y will have the opportunity then to present her case. Also, the patient care record and testimony of others in the clinic about customary practice will provide evidence as to causation.

Y was also astute to avoid arguing with patient X about possible contributory negligence in failing to alert Y that he was burning, etc. Y displayed a caring, concerned attitude for patient X's welfare and obtained appropriate follow-up care for him. That empathetic intervention alone may prevent a claim from ever being filed.

A concomitant patient care progress note entry for patient X might read:

> Sept. 19, 201x/1415 hours: 1 7/8-in.-diameter round erythematous dry blister noted at patient's R A-C jt prior to rx. Notified Mary Therapist, P.T., who examined pt. and ordered rx. withheld until examination by Dr. S. Follow-up pending.

2. The examining physician should consider the possibility that patient C is the victim of elder abuse. Patient C displays many of the classic signs of possible abuse, including physical symptoms that do not necessarily conform to the attributed source of injury, withdrawal in the face of questions about her injuries, inappropriate dress for the season, pain symptoms distant from the injury site (shoulders), general deconditioning, a reported history of repetitive falling, and a family member answering questions for her without apparent need. The intern should consult with the facility risk manager and/or legal advisor to ascertain any mandatory reporting requirements and coordinate with social services for further social intervention. The physician should carefully document objective evaluative (including radiologic) findings and transcribe verbatim any statements patient C might make concerning attribution of her injuries. Patient C's record should

receive special handling, and her case should be reviewed expeditiously for the need for reporting and/or further intervention.

REVIEW ACTIVITIES

1. Develop a brief (50-word or less) patients' written acknowledgment of receipt of a Patient Notice of Privacy Practices (in English and Spanish) that is required to be issued to patients on their first visit to a HIPAA-covered entity clinic.

2. Develop an elective informed consent form for use and disclosure by a HIPAA-covered entity clinic of a patient's PHI for purposes of treatment, payment for services and administrative operations of the business without further patient authorization or consent (so called *routine uses*).

Epilogue

Although the ethical, legal and practical patient care documentation-related obligations incumbent upon healthcare professionals are many and complex, they can be better understood through education, and, as a result, providers can have greater peace of mind while they carry out documentation tasks related to care-related activities performed on behalf of patients.

These are the principle purposes of this book: to educate healthcare professionals about key ethical, legal, and practical aspects of patient care documentation, so that they may be the best fiduciaries possible to patients under their care; to make them aware of their legal rights and duties incident to patient care documentation; to give them a framework to assess their official documentation-related conduct for compliance with competency, customary, ethical, and legal standards; and to provide them with the tools to practice effective liability risk management associated with patient care documentation.

Because patient care documentation standards and methods are ever evolving, readers are urged to involve administrators, attorneys, ethicists, information management specialists, and relevant others in their practices and continuing education experiences. Through optimal patient care documentation methods and management, healthcare professionals will simultaneously protect the vital interests of their patients and themselves.

Glossary of Legal Terms

Abandonment—A situation in which a healthcare provider improperly unilaterally terminates a professional relationship with a patient.

Advance directives—Legal instruments that memorialize patient desires concerning life-sustaining measures to be taken and decision making should the patient subsequently become legally incapacitated (e.g., living will, durable power of attorney for healthcare decision-making, out-of-facility do not resuscitate order, and declaration for mental health treatment).

Apparent agency—A situation in which a court will impose vicarious liability on an employer for the actions of a contractor working for the employer because the contractor is indistinguishable from an employee in the eyes of the public.

Assault—The apprehension or anticipation of the application of unauthorized physical force.

Attorney work product—Documentation prepared on a client's behalf in anticipation of litigation.

Attorney–client privilege—In the law of evidence, a client's privilege to refuse to disclose, and to prevent any other person from disclosing, confidential communications between the client and his/her attorney.

Autonomy—Self-determination.

Battery—The unconsented, unprivileged harmful or offensive touching of another person.

Beneficence—Acting in patients' best interests.

Beyond a reasonable doubt—The standard (burden) of proof in a criminal case, by which the government must prove a criminal defendant's guilt to the satisfaction of a jury or judge.

Business associate—A person who, on behalf of a covered entity, provides legal services involving the disclosure of individually identifiable health information.

Collateral source rule—A legal rule related to (money) damages determination in a civil case under which a jury is prevented from knowing about a plaintiff's collateral sources of recovery for injuries, such as insurance payments and partial payments in settlement from other defendants in the case.

Comparative fault—Consideration by a judge or jury, not just of a defendant's conduct, but also that of the plaintiff in a civil lawsuit. If the plaintiff failed to exercise that degree of reasonable care expected by society to protect oneself from harm, the plaintiff's (money) damages for injury at the defendant's hands may be reduced or even eliminated.

Compensatory damages—Money awarded by a court to a tort plaintiff to make the plaintiff "whole," such as for lost wages or salary (present and future), medical expenses (present and future), pain and suffering, and loss of enjoyment of life.

Complaint—A formal legal document specifying an incident allegedly causing patient-plaintiff injury and the amount of (money) damages sought.

Confidential—Knowledge or document deemed as sensitive.

Conspiracy—A situation in which two or more people agree to commit an unlawful act. When charged as a criminal action, it is a separate offense from any underlying crime (e.g., fraud, obstruction of justice, or perjury).

Corporate liability—Under law, hospitals and private clinics have certain responsibilities that they may not delegate to employees, professional medical staff, or independent contractors.

Crime—A tort that is a public action or wrong against society as a whole.

Criminal action—Public action brought by the government for a wrong or wrongs against society as a whole.

Cross-examination—In court, questions by the opposition after a witness has testified on direct examination.

Defamation—A communication to a third party on an untrue statement about a person that damages the defamed person's good reputation in the community. Two classifications of defamation are slander (oral defamation) and libel (written or other forms of defamation).

Deponent—A person undergoing deposition.

Deposition—A pretrial "discovery" device consisting of sworn testimony of a party or potential party to a lawsuit, or of a fact or expert witness.

Directed verdict—A situation in which the party with the burden to prove a legal case fails to present a prima facie case (i.e., one on which the party could prevail), requiring the judge to refuse to allow the case to go to the jury for its consideration.

Discovery—A phase of the pretrial process where experts and those involved in a lawsuit answer questions in interviews or under oath in depositions by one or both parties in a case.

Durable power of attorney for health care—A legal document, signed by a patient, that delegates healthcare treatment decision making to an agent of the patient's choice in the event that the patient becomes legally incompetent.

Emergency doctrine—An exception to the requirement to obtain patient informed consent before treatment for emergency lifesaving care.

Exculpatory contract—A contract between a patient and healthcare provider in which the provider attempts to limit or eliminate his or her liability for ordinary or professional negligence incident to care.

Expert witness—A witness possessing expertise concerning a relevant issue in a legal case, based on special knowledge, skill, and/or training.

Fact witness—Also called a "percipient" witness or eyewitness, one who possesses relevant firsthand knowledge about the issues and merits of a legal case important to one or both sides.

Fiduciaries—Persons and entities in a special position of trust (e.g., relationship between healthcare professionals and entities with their patients).

Fiduciary relationship—A special relationship in which a trustee is expected to put the interests of a beneficiary ahead of his or her own personal interests.

FMEA: failure mode and effect analysis—A quality management tool and systematic procedure utilized to rank and prioritize possible causes of product failure and to implement preventive measures.

Fraud—A false representation of material (decisional) fact, made with the intent to deceive, which causes another person to take some action detrimental to his or her own (or the public's) interest.

Healthcare malpractice—An adverse outcome (injury) associated with patient treatment, coupled with a recognized basis for imposing liability, such as professional negligence, failure to achieve a therapeutic promise (breach of contract), or injury from a dangerously defective product (product liability).

Healthcare "malpractice crisis"—Characterized by a public perception of increasing numbers of legal actions and larger civil malpractice verdicts in favor of patient-plaintiffs and against defendant–healthcare providers and organizations, all of which overwhelm the U.S. legal system.

Hearsay—Any out-of-court statement offered as evidence in court for the truth of the matter asserted in it; describes secondhand input; a patient's extemporaneous "excited utterances" transcribed in the patient care record.

HIPAA—The Health Insurance Portability and Accountability Act of 1996, a federal statute with several key purposes: to make employee health insurance benefits portable from job to job, to safeguard patient health information privacy, and to streamline electronic third-party billing procedures.

Independent contractor—A worker for whom an employer normally is not vicariously liable, based primarily on the lack of control over the physical details of the contractor's work product.

Inference—A trial rule that allows, but does not compel, a conclusion of negligence by a jury based on permissive deductive reasoning.

Informed consent—Providing a patient with sufficient information about a proposed treatment and its reasonable alternatives to allow the patient to make a knowing, intelligent, and unequivocal decision regarding whether to accept or reject the proposed treatment.

Informed refusal—A decision by the patient to refuse care after the informed consent process, and after a provider has explained objectively the expected consequences of refusing examination and/or intervention.

Intentional abandonment—Abrupt discharge of a patient for reasons such as failure to pay a bill, a personality conflict with a treating healthcare professional, or an insurance denial of reimbursement for further care without the provider notifying the patient of an intent to terminate, and giving enough time for the patient to find another healthcare provider or helping him or her to find an alternate care provider, etc. (see, patient abandonment).

Intentional misconduct—A potential exception to vicarious liability; an act committed by an employee that is considered on a case by case basis to consider whether the employer undertook all available reasonable steps to ensure patient safety.

Interrogatories—Formal written pretrial "discovery" questions posed by one party in a civil case to another, for which answers are required.

Invasion of privacy—An intentional tort that involves the public disclosure of private facts; intentional dissemination of private information about a person to a third party not having a legal right to know the information revealed.

Joint and several liability—Among more than one defendant possibly liable to a plaintiff for injury, personal individual responsibility of each defendant for the whole amount of the plaintiff's damages.

Jurisdiction—A court's legal authority to hear a specific legal case and exercise control over the parties.

Larceny by fraud—Theft of money, goods, services, or other property by deception.

Libel—Written defamatory remarks about another person; also includes defamatory statements made on computer, videotape, or other relatively permanent media (*see*, defamation).

Living will—A legal document, signed by a patient, that states the patient's desires regarding lifesustaining measures to be taken in the event that the patient becomes legally incompetent.

Managed care—The current predominant healthcare delivery and reimbursement paradigm under which cost containment is at least as important as patient welfare and quality care delivery.

Measuring and evaluating patient care (M & E)—The systematic evaluation of selected clinical indicators concerning important aspects of patient care as part of a program to improve quality or organizational performance.

National Practitioner Data Bank—A federal database maintained under private contract for the Department of Health and Human Services to store information concerning adverse licensure, privileging, and malpractice payments involving licensed healthcare providers.

Negligent abandonment—A type of malpractice action where the patient claims that he or she was discharged prematurely.

Nondelegable duties—Duties owed directly by a healthcare facility to its patients, including the duty to select and retain only competent healthcare providers, the duty to maintain safe premises and equipment, and the duty to oversee the quality of patient care provided in the facility.

Nonmaleficence—Do no malicious intentional harm.

Obstruction of justice—Intentionally altering or destroying records or other relevant material to eliminate or distort the true account of an event.

Patient abandonment—Legally actionable; occurs when a healthcare provider improperly unilaterally terminates a professional relationship with a patient (*see*, professional negligence, intentional misconduct).

Patient care record—A memorialization of a specific patient's health status at a given point in time, and over an extended time period that serves as a business document and as the legal record of care rendered to the patient.

Partnership vicarious liability—Where each partner normally is vicariously liable or indirectly financially responsible for the other partners' negligent acts or omissions committed within the scope of activities of the partnership.

Phantom billing—Fraudulent filing of claims for health professional services not actually rendered.

Premises liability—The legal duties of a landowner or occupier to maintain premises that are safe for business visitors and others, as determined by applicable state law.

Preponderance of evidence—The usual standard (burden) of proof in a civil case, in which the party with the burden (usually the plaintiff [party bringing suit]) must prove his or her case by a greater weight of evidence.

Present recollection refreshed—The use of hearsay evidence in court to remind a witness of events is called *present recollection refreshed*.

Presumption—A trial rule that requires a jury to presume negligence against a defendant unless and until the defendant introduces sufficient evidence to rebut the presumption.

Private action—A tort involving injuries personal to private parties.

Pro bon publico—The rendition of free of charge or reduced fee services to clients lacking the ability to pay full market value for them.

Professional negligence—Delivery of patient care that falls below the standard expected of ordinary reasonable practitioners of the same profession acting under the same or similar circumstances.

Punitive damages—Punishment damages imposed upon a civil defendant when the defendant's conduct is deemed egregious.

Quality management—A global concept that includes development, implementation, monitoring, analysis, and revision, as needed, of information, liability-avoidance, patient care, and resource utilization healthcare delivery systems.

Request for admission—A legal tool used to validate a document as genuine or admit/deny the truth of a statement; used at the end of the discovery process of a trial to settle uncontested issues or the trial itself (*see,* discovery).

Res ipsa loquitur—Latin for "the thing speaks for itself." Under this legal doctrine, a patient-plaintiff 's burden of proof may be lessened if (1) the patient's injury was the kind that normally does not occur absent negligence, (2) the defendant-provider exercised exclusive control over the treatment or modality that caused the patient injury, and (3) the patient was not contributorily negligent.

Risk management—The process of systematically monitoring healthcare delivery activities in order to prevent or minimize financial losses from claims or lawsuits arising from patient care or other activities conducted in a healthcare facility.

Routine uses—Use and disclosure by a covered entity of a patient's PHI for purposes of treatment, payment for services, and internal healthcare operations of the business, without the patient's authorization or consent.

Sexual battery—The unconsented, unprivileged harmful or offensive touching of the sexual or other intimate parts of another person, for the purpose of sexual arousal (of either party), gratification, or abuse.

Slander—Spoken defamatory remarks (*see,* defamation).

Spoliation—The intentional wrongful destruction or alteration of a document, done for the purpose of changing or concealing its original meaning.

Standard of care—The benchmark delineating nonnegligent and negligent patient care, a defendant's (party being sued) professional conduct is compared to that of ordinary reasonable peers acting under the same or similar circumstances.

Statement against interest—An out-of-court statement made by a person that is against the declarant's own pecuniary or proprietary interests. A statement against one's own interests is admissible in court as an exception to the hearsay rule.

Statute of limitations—A "time clock" for initiating a lawsuit, after the expiration of which further relief is forever time barred.

Statutes of repose—Absolute time limits within which legal action must be commenced.

Subpoena duces tecum—A court order to the custodian of documents or other things that are pertinent to issues in a legal case to deliver them for inspection to a business location or to bring them when testifying at a legal proceeding, such as a pretrial deposition or a trial.

Summary judgment—Granting a court verdict in favor of a party to the case without a trial, when the pretrial documents demonstrate that there are no material issues of fact to decide by resort to trial.

Summons—Formal notification of a lawsuit.

Technicality—Refers to a detail of the law that results in a legal decision or verdict.

Telehealth—Computerized information transfer systems and technology used to transmit patient care and related data to distant providers having a need for the information conveyed.

Therapeutic privilege—Where a healthcare provider may be excused from disclosing information to a patient who, in the provider's professional judgment, could not psychologically cope with the information disclosed.

Tolled—An interruption in the statutes of limitations.

Tort—(French, meaning "wrongs") A class of civil legal actions that includes most private injuries except breach of contract actions.

Tort reform—Legislative and judicial action undertaken in recent decades to decrease the number of tort lawsuits.

Tortfeasor—Wrongdoer

Total quality management—A strategic integrated management system for achieving client/customer/patient satisfaction, which involves all managers and employees, anduses quantitative methods to help improve an organization's processes.

Unbundling—Overutilization of healthcare-related products and services paid for by third-party payers; a type of fraud.

Unintentional misconduct—A potential exception to vicarious liability; an act committed by an employee that is considered on a case-by-case basis to consider whether the employer undertook all available reasonable steps to ensure patient safety.

Upcoding—Fraudulent miscategorizing of procedural terminology codes to enhance reimbursement.

Vicarious liability—(also, *respondeat superior* [Latin for "let the master answer"]) Indirect financial responsibility for the conduct of another person, usually an employee acting within the scope of his or her employment.

Acronyms

AARA	American Recovery and Reinvestment Act
ADL	activities of daily living
AHRQ	Agency for Healthcare Research and Quality
CARF	Commission on Accreditation of Rehabilitation Facilities
CMS	Center for Medicare Services
CPRS	Computerized Medical Records System (Veteran's Administration)
CPT-4	*Current Procedural Terminology*, 4th edition
DNR	do-not-resuscitate (orders)
EHRs	electronic health records
EMR	electronic medical records
FMEA	failure mode and effect analysis
HEDIS	Health Plan Employer Data and Information Set
HHA	home health agency
HPSAs	health professional shortage areas
ICD-9	*International Classification of Diseases*, 9th edition
JC	Joint Commission (National Committee on Quality Assurance)
LTG	long-term (ADL) goals
NCQA	National Committee on Quality Assurance
OASIS-C	Outcome and Assessment Information Set
OCR	Office of Civil Rights
OSHA	Occupational Safety and Health Administration
PCE	potentially compensable event
PHI	protected health information

POMR	problem-oriented medical record system
PSP	problem–status–plan
QI	quality insurance
RBRVS	Resource-Based Relative Value System (CMS)
SNF	skilled nursing facility
SOAP	subjective, objective, assessment, and plan
SOAPG	subjective, objective, assessment, plan, and interventional goals
STG	short-term (ADL) goals
TPO	treatment, payment, and operations (permissive disclosures, HIPAA)
TQM	total quality management
VistA	Veterans Health Information Systems and Technology Architecture

Example of a Representative Abbreviation List for a Rehabilitation Service

Note: While the trend in health care is away from overusing abbreviations in patient care documentation—especially confusing ones like "q.d.", "q.i.d.", and "q.o.d."—they remain useful, when used sparingly, and when their meaning is universally understood. The following is a sample list of abbreviations that might be used in a physical rehabilitation facility.

A

A–active, artery, assessment

A/–before

AA–active assist, arteries, Alcoholics Anonymous

AAA–abdominal aortic aneurysm

AAROM–active-assisted range of motion

AB–abortion, antibiotics

ABD–abdominal, abduction

ABG–arterial blood gasses

ABN–abnormal

ABO–blood grouping system

AC–acromioclavicular, alternating current, anterior cruciate, assisted control (ventilation), before meals (ante cibum)

ACJ–acromioclavicular joint

ACL–anterior cruciate ligament

ACLR–anterior cruciate ligament reconstruction
ACT–active
ADD–adduction
ADH–antidiuretic hormone
ADL–activities of daily living
AD LIB–as desired
ADM–admission
AE–above elbow
AER–aerosol
AF–atrial fibrillation, anterior fontanel
AFO–ankle-foot orthosis
AFS–assessment flow sheet
AGA–appropriate for gestational age
AHF–antihemophilic factor
AI–aortic insufficiency
AIDS–acquired immunodeficiency syndrome
AIIS–anterior inferior iliac spine
AJ–ankle jerk
AKA–above knee amputation
ALB–albumin
ALTE–apparent life-threatening event
AMA–against medical advice
AMB–ambulation
AMP–ampule
ANT–anterior
AN–antigen
ANES–anesthesia
ANT–anterior
A&O–alert and oriented
AODM–adult-onset diabetes mellitus
AP–ankle pumps, anterior-posterior
APC–atrial premature contraction
AR–aortic regurgitation
ARDS–acute respiratory distress syndrome
ARF–acute renal failure
AROM–active range of motion
ASA–aspirin
ASAP–as soon as possible

ASCAD–atherosclerotic coronary artery disease
ASD–atrial septal defect
ASHD–arteriosclerotic heart disease
ASIS–anterior superior iliac spine
AS TOL–as tolerated
ATFL–anterior talofibular ligament
AVM–arteriovenous malformation
AVN–avascular necrosis
AVR–aortic valve replacement

B

B–bilateral
BA swallow–Barium swallow
BAB–Babinski sign
BASO–basophil
BB–back bending
BBB–bundle branch block
BC–blood culture
BDAE–Boston Diagnostic Aphasia Evaluation
BE–below elbow, Barium enema
BID–twice daily
BIL–bilateral
BILI–bilirubin
BIW–twice weekly
BK–below the knee
BKA–below-knee amputation
BLA–baseline assessment
BLAD–bladder
BLE–bilateral lower extremities
BM–bowel movement, breast milk
BMT–bone marrow transplant
BP–blood pressure
BPD–bronchopulmonary dysplagia
BPM–beats per minute
BR–breast
BRACH–brachial
BRONCH–bronchoscopy
BRP–bathroom privileges

BS–bedside, bowel sounds, breath sounds

B-STREP–beta hemolytic strep

BSO–bilateral salpingo-oophorectomy

BTB–bone-tendon-bone

BTL–bilateral tubal ligation

BTU–British thermal unit

BUE–bilateral upper extremities

BUN–blood urea nitrogen

BW–birth weight, body weight

BX–biopsy

C

C–cervical

C/–with C1, 2 . . . 7–cervical spinal levels

C&S–culture and sensitivity

CA–calcium, cancer, coronary artery

CABG–coronary artery bypass graft

3VCABG—three-vessel coronary artery bypass graft

CAD–coronary artery disease

CAL–calorie

CAP–capillary

CAPD–continuous ambulatory peritoneal dialysis

CARF–Commission on Accreditation of Rehabilitation Facilities

CATH–cardiac catheterization

CBC–complete blood count

CBD–common bile duct

CBI–continuous bladder irrigation

CBS–chronic brain syndrome

CC–chief complaint, cubic centimeter

CCU–cardiac/constant care unit

CDH–congenital diaphragmatic hernia

CEA–carotid enarterotomy

CFL–calcaneofibular ligament

CHF–congestive heart failure

CHI–closed head injury

CHO–carbohydrates

CHR–chronic

CL–chlorine

CLAV–clavicle

CLD–chronic lung disease

CM–centimeter

CMP–chondromalacia patella

CMS–Center for Medicare and Medicaid Services (formerly HCFA)

CMV–cytomegalovirus

CN–cranial nerve

CNS–central nervous system

CO–cardiac output

C/O–complains of

COG DEF–cognitive deficit(s)

COGN–cognitive

COLD–chronic obstructive lung disease

CONT–continue(s), continue(d)

COPD–chronic obstructive pulmonary disease

CORT–certified operating room technician

COTA–certified occupational therapist assistant

CP–calf pumps, cerebral palsy, chest pain, cold pack

CPK–creatinine phosphokinase

CPM–continuous passive motion

CPR–cardiopulmonary resuscitation

CPS–Child Protective Services

CPT–chest physical therapy

CR–crutch(es), cardiorespiratory

CRF–chronic renal failure

CRI–chronic renal insufficiency

CRNP–certified registered nurse practitioner

CS–Caesarian section

CSF–cerebrospinal fluid

CSM–circulatory, sensory, motor

CT–computerized tomography, cholecystectomy tube

CTN–contraction

CTR–carpal tunnel release

CTS–cardiothoracic surgery, carpal tunnel syndrome

CV–cardiovascular

CVA–cerebral vascular accident, costovertebral angle

CVP–central venous pressure

CVT–cardiovascular technologist

CW–crutch walking (NWB: nonweight bearing; TWB: touch weight bearing; PWB: partial weight bearing; WBAT: weight bearing as tolerated; FWB: full weight bearing)

CWI–crutch walking instruction
CX–cervical
CXR–chest X-ray
CYSTO–cystoscopy

D

D–dorsal, distal
D/3–distal one third
DA–developmental age
DC–Doctor of Chiropractic
D/C–direct current, discontinue
D&C–dilation and curretage
DDD–degenerative disc disease
DDS–Doctor of Dental Surgery
DEC–decrease(d)
DEP–dependent
DEPT–department
DF–dorsiflexion
DIP–distal interphalangeal joint
DIST–distal
DJD–degenerative joint disease
DM–diabetes mellitus
DNK–did not keep (appointment)
DO–doctor of osteopathy
DOA–date of admission, dead on arrival
DOE–dyspnea on exertion
DOI–date of injury
DON–Department of Nursing
DOS–date of surgery
DPC–delayed primary closure
DPT–diphtheria, pertussis, tetanus
DT–delirium tremens
DTD–dated
DTR–deep tendon reflex
DUB–dysfunctional uterine bleeding
DVT–deep vein thrombosis
DX–diagnosis

E

EA–educational age

EAD–end artery disease

EBV–Epstein-Barr virus

ECF–extended care facility

ECG (or EKG)–electrocardiogram

ECHO–echocardiogram

ECMO–extracorporeal membrane oxygenation

E coli–*Escherichia coli*

ED–Emergency Department

EDX–electrodiagnosis

EEG–electroencephalogram

EENT–eye, ear, nose, and throat

EHR–exercise heart rate

EIL–extension in lying

EIS–extension in standing

ELEV–elevated

EMG–electromyogram

EOS–Eosinophils

EOSS–end-of-shift summation

EPITH–epithelium

ER–emergency room, external rotation

ES–electrostimulation

ESR–Erythrocyte Sedimentation Rate

ESRD–end-stage renal disease

ET–endothracheal

ETIOL–etiology

ETOH–ethanol

ETT–endotracheal tube

EV–eversion

EX–exercise

EXPIR–expiration

EXT–extension, external, extract, extremity

F

F–fair (muscle test grade), female

FAB ER–flexion/abduction/external rotation

FAROM–full active range of motion

FB–foreign body, forward bending

F/B–followed by

FBS–fasting blood sugar

FCE–functional capacity evaluation

FE–iron

FES–functional electric stimulation

FFAROM–full functional active range of motion

FFP–fresh-frozen plasma

FH–family history

FHM–fetal heart monitor(ing)

FHS–family health services

FHT–fetal heart tones

FIB–fibula

FIL–flexion in lying

FIS–flexion in standing

FLEX–flexion

FMEA–failure mode and effect analysis

FOOSH–fall onto outstretched hand

FPROM–full passive range of motion

FREQ–frequency, frequent

FSH–Follicle Stimulating Hormone

FT–feet, foot

FTN–finger-to-nose

FTP–failure to progress

FTSG–full-thickness skin graft

FTT–failure to thrive

F/U–follow-up

FUB–functional uterine bleeding

FUO–fever of unknown origin

FVC–forced vital capacity

FWB–full weight bearing

FX–fracture

G

G–good (muscle test grade), gravida

GA–gestational age

GB–gallbladder

GC–*Gonococcus*

GCS–Glasgow Coma Scale

GE–gastroenterology

GEL–gelatin

GETA–general endotracheal anesthesia

GI–gastrointestinal

GLOB–globulin

GM–gram

GMO–general medical officer

GMT–gross muscle test

GN–graduate nurse

GP(FP)AL–gravida (number of pregnancies), para (number of pregnancies resulting in live offspring), (number of deliveries at full term, number of premature deliveries), number of abortions (elective or spontaneous), number of living offspring

GS–gluteal setting

GSW–gunshot wound

GT–drops, gait training

GTT–glucose tolerance test

GU–genitourinary

GYN–gynecology

H

H–hemovac

H & H–hemoglobin and hematocrit

H & P–history and physical exam

HA–headache

HB, HGB–hemoglobin

HBIG–hepatitis-B immune globulin

HBP–high blood pressure

HC–head circumference, hydrocephalus, hydrocortisone

HCFA–Health Care Financing Administration (now CMS)

HCG–human chorionic gonadotrophin

HCL–hydrochloric acid

HCP–hydrocortisone phonophoresis

HCT–hematocrit

HCV–hepatitis-C virus

HCVD–hypertensive cardiovascular disease

HEDIS–Health Employers Data Information Set [for HMOs]
HEENT–head, eyes, ears, nose, throat
HEMI–hemiplegic
HFO–high frequency oscillation
HFPP–high frequency positive pressure (ventilation)
HGH–human growth hormone
HI–head injury
HIPAA–Health Insurance Portability and Accountability Act of 1996
HIS–hospital information system
HIV–human immunodeficiency virus
HMO–health maintenance organization
HNP–herniated nucleus pulposus
HOB–head of bed
HOC–head-on collision
HOH–hard of hearing
HOSP–hospital
HP–hot pack, home program
HPI–history of present illness
HPV–human papilloma virus
HR–heart rate, hour(s)
HS–hamstring muscles, hour of sleep (horasomni)
HSM–hepatosplenomegaly
HSS–hamstring sets (isometric exercise)
HSV–herpes simplex virus
HT–height, Hubbard tank
HTN–hypertension
HVD–hypertensive vascular disease
HVGS–high-voltage galvanic stimulation
HX–history
HYPO–hypodermic

I

I–independent
I & D–incision and drainage
I&O–intake and output
IBW–ideal body weight
IC or I/C–informed consent
ICB–intracranial bleeding

ICF–immediate care facility

ICH–intracerebral hemorrhage

ICP–intracranial pressure

ICT–intermittent cervical traction

ICU–intensive care unit

ID–infectious disease

IDDM–insulin-dependent diabetes mellitus

IDK–internal derangement of the knee

IDM–infant of a diabetic mother

IFES–interferential electric stimulation

IH–infectious hepatitis

II–image intensifier

IM–ice massage, intermuscular (injection)

IMCN–intermediate care nursery

IMI–inferior myocardial infarction

IMP–impairment, impression

IN–inch(es)

INC–incontinent, increase(d)

INF–inferior

IN SITU–in natural position

INT–intact, internal

INV–inversion

IP–interphalangeal

IPPB–intermittent positive pressure breathing

IPT–intermittent pelvic traction

IR–internal rotation

IRREG–irregular

IS–incentive spirometry

ISO–isoenzyme

ISS–injury severity score

IU–international units

IUD–intrauterine device

IV–intravenous

IVC–inferior vena cava

IVF–intravenous fluid

IVH–intraventricular hemorrhage

IVP–intravenous pyelogram

IVSD–intraventricular septal defect

J

JCAHO–Joint Commission on Accreditation of Healthcare Organizations
JRA–juvenile rheumatoid arthritis
JT–joint

K

K–potassium
KAFO–knee-ankle-foot orthosis
KCAL–kilocalories
KG–kilogram
KJ–knee jerk
KUB–kidney/ureter/bladder

L

L–length, left, liter, lumbar
L1, 2 . . . 5–lumbar spinal levels
L/3–lower one-third
LA–left atrium
L&A–light and accommodation
LAC–laceration(s), long arm cast
LACR–lacrimation
LAMI–laminectomy
LAP–laparotomy
LAT–lateral, latissimus dorsi muscle
LAV–lavatory
LB–low back, pound
LBBB–left bundle branch block
LBP–low back pain
LBW–low birth weight
LC–living children
LCL–lateral collateral ligament
LE–lower extremity
LEUC–leukocyte
LFC–lateral femoral condyle
LGA–large for gestational age
LGE–large
LIG–ligament

LL–left lumbar (scoliosis)

LLC–long leg cast

LLE–left lower extremity

LLL–left lower lobe (of lung)

LLWC–long leg walking cast

LMN–lower motor neuron

LMP–last menstrual period

LMT–lateral meniscus tear

LOC–loss of consciousness

LOM–loss of motion

LOS–length of stay

LP–lumbar puncture

LPM–liters per minute

LPN–licensed practical nurse

LRQ–lower right quadrant

LS–lumbosacral

LT–left, left thoracic (scoliosis), Levin tube

LTG–long-term goal(s)

LTM–long-term memory

LUE–left upper extremity

LUQ–left upper quadrant

LV–left ventricle

LVE–left ventricular enlargement

LVH–left ventricular hypertrophy

LYM–lymphocyte

LYTE–electrolyte

M

M–meter, male

M/3–middle one-third

MA–medical assistance

MA–milliamperes

MAE–moves all extremities

MAMMO–mammogram

MAP–mean airway pressure

MASS–massage

MAX–maximum

MC–managed care, Medicare

MCA–motorcycle accident

MCL–medial collateral ligament

MCP–metacarpophalangeal

MCTD–mixed connective tissue disease

MD–medical doctor, muscular dystrophy

MDI–metered dose inhaler

MED–medical, medication(s)

MEDCO–medcollator

MEDSON–medsonalator

MEQ–milliequivalents

METS–metastases

MFC–medial femoral condyle

MG–milligram, myasethenia gravis

MH–moist heat

MI–myocardial infarction

MICU–medical intensive care unit

MID–middle, midline

MIN–minimum, minute(s)

ML–milliliter

MM–millimeter, meningomyelocele, muscle(s)

MMAI–maximal multiple angle isometrics

MMT–manual muscle test

MO–month(s)

MOD–moderate, modified

MOM–milk of magnesia

MONO–monocyte

MPS–multiphasis screening

MR–mitral regurgitation

MRI–magnetic resonance imaging

MRM–modified radical mastectomy

MRN–medical record number

MS–multiple sclerosis

MSR–muscle stretch reflex

MT–manual (or manipulative) therapy, medical technologist

MTF–medical treatment facility, medial tibial flare

MTP–metatarsophalangeal

MV–millivolt
MVA–motor vehicle accident
MVR–mitral valve replacement
MVT–movement
MYELO–myeolgram

N

N–normal (muscle test grade), nitrogen
N/A–not applicable
NAD–no apparent distress
NAR–no apparent reason (or rationale)
NAS–no added salt
NB–newborn
NC–nasal cannula, no change
NCQA–National Committee on Quality Assurance
NCV–nerve conduction velocity
NDB–nursing database
NDT–neurodevelopmental treatment
NEG–negative
NF–National Formulary
NG–nasogastric
NH–nursing home
NHP–nursing home placement
NICU–neonatal intensive care unit
NIDDM–non-insulin-dependent diabetes mellitus
NKA–no known allergies
NKI–no known illnesses/injuries
NL–normal (limits)
NN–nerve(s)
NO, #–number
NOC–night, nightly
N–p–nasopharyngeal
NPO–nothing by mouth (nil per os)
NQWMI–non-Q wave myocardial infarction
NSAID–nonsteroidal anti-inflammatory drug
NSR–normal sinus rhythm
NSS–newborn supplemental screening

NSVD–normal spontaneous vaginal delivery

NTG–nitroglycerine

NWB–nonweight bearing

O

O–objective

OASIS–Outcome and Assessment Information Set (Medicare home health assessment instrument)

OB–obstetrics, occult blood

OBS–organic brain syndrome

OCT–oxytocin

OD–once daily, overdose, right eye, doctor of optometry

OM–oral motor

OME–oral motor exercise

OOB–out of bed

OOP–out of plaster

OP–outpatient

O&P–ova and parasites

OPD–outpatient department

OPR–outpatient record

OPV–oral polio vaccine

OR–operating room

ORIF–open reduction internal fixation

OS–left eye

OT–occupational therapist/therapy

OTO–otology

OTR–registered occupational therapist

OX–oximetery

OZ–ounce

P

P–para, plan, poor (muscle test grade), pulse

P/–after

P/3–proximal one third

PA–physician assistant, posterior-anterior

P&A–percussion and auscultation

PAC–premature atrial contraction

PAF–paroxysmal atrial fibrillation

PALP–palpation
PARA–paraplegic
PAT–paroxysmal atrial tachycardia, pre-admission testing
PATH–pathology
PAW–pulmonary artery wedge pressure
PB–lead, periodic breathing
PC–after meals
PCA–patient-controlled anesthesia
PCG–pneumocardiogram
PCL–posterior cruciate ligament
PCV–packed cell volume
PDP–postural drainage and percussion
PDR–*Physician's Desk Reference*
PE–physical examination, pulmonary embolus
PEEP–positive end expiratory pressure
PED–pediatric
PEN–penicillin
PER–by
PERRLA–pupils equal, round, reactive to light and accommodation
PF–peak flow, plantar flexion
PFJS–patellofemoral joint syndrome
PFR–peak flow rate
PFT–pulmonary function test
PGH–pituitary growth hormone
PH–past history
PID–pelvic inflammatory disease
PIE–pulmonary interstitial emphysema
PINS–posterior interosseous nerve syndrome
PIP–peak inspiratory pressure, proximal interphalangeal joint
PMH–past medical history
PMI–point of maximal intensity, posterior myocardial infarction
PMR–physical medicine and rehabilitation
PMS–physical medicine service
PND–paroxysmal nocturnal dyspnea
PNF–proprioceptive neuromuscular facilitation
PNI–peripheral nerve injury
PO–by mouth (per os)
POC–products of conception

POMR–problem-oriented medical record

POS–positive

POSS–possible

POST–posterior

POST-OP–after surgery

POX–pulse oximtery

PPB–positive pressure breathing

PPN–peripheral parenteral nutrition

PPO–preferred provider organization

PPS–prospective payment system

PRE–progressive resistive exercises

PRE-OP–before surgery

PREP–prepare for

PRM–premature rupture of membranes

PRN–whenever needed

PROB–problem, probable

PROG–progress

PROM–passive range of motion

PRON–pronation

PROX–proximal

PSIS–posterior superior iliac spine

PT–patient, physical therapy, physical training, pint, point, prothrombin time

PTA–physical therapist assistant, prior to admission

PTB–patellar tendon bearing

PTCA–percutaneous transluminal coronary angioplasty

PTFL–posterior talofibular ligament

PTL–pre-term labor

PTP–patient teaching protocol

PUD–peptic ulcer disease

PV–post-voiding

PVC–premature ventricular contraction

PVD–peripheral vascular disease

PVR–pulmonary vascular resistance

Q

Q–every (quaque)

QA–quality assurance

QD–every day

Q4HR–every 4 hours
QH–every hour
QI–quality improvement
QID–four times a day
QIP–quality improvement program
QIT–quality improvement team
QN–very night
QOD–every other day
QRS–ventricular complex (on ECG)
QS–quadriceps muscle sets, quantity sufficient
QUAD–quadriceps muscles, quadriplegic

R

R–respirations, right
RA–rheumatoid arthritis, right atrium
RBA–risks, benefits, (reasonable) alternatives
RBC–red blood cell (count)
RCR–rotator cuff repair
RCS–rotator cuff strain
RCT–rotator cuff tear
RD–radial deviation, registered dietician
RDS–respiratory distress syndrome
RE–recheck, regarding
RE-ADM–readmission
RE-ED–re-education
REP–repetition(s)
RESP–respiratory
RH–Rhesus factor
RHD–rheumatic heart disease
RHR–resting heart rate
RL–right lumbar (scoliosis)
RLE–right lower extremity
RLQ–right lower quadrant
RN–registered nurse
RNC–registered nurse certified
RND–radical neck dissection
R/O–rule out
ROM–range of motion, rupture of membranes

ROS–review of systems
RPPS–retropatellar pain syndrome
RR–respiratory rate
RRA–registered record administrator
RSLR–reverse straight leg raise
RST–restart
RT–right, radiation therapy, right thoracic (scoliosis)
RTC–return to clinic
RTR–registered technologist radiology
RTW–return to work
RUE–right upper extremity
RUL–right upper lobe (of lung)
RV–right ventricle
RX–treatment, prescription

S

S–sacral, supervision
S/–without
SS–one-half (semsis)
SA–sino-atrial node
SAA–same as above
SAB–spontaneous abortion
SAC–short arm cast
SACH–solid ankle cushion heel
SAH–subarachnoid hemorrhage
SAHS–short-arc hamstring (exercise)
SAQ–short-arc quad (triceps exercise)
SB–side-bending
SBE–subacute bacterial endocarditis
SBQC–small-based quad cane
SC–subcutaneous
SCAP–scapula(r)
SCFE–slipped capital femoral epiphysis
SCI–spinal cord injury
SCJ–sternoclavicular joint
SCM–sternocleidomastoid
SCP–standard care plan
SD–septal defect

SDH–subdural hematoma

SEC–second(s)

SED RATE–sedimentation rate

SEGS–segmented neutrophils

SEM VES–seminal vesicles

SF–synovial fluid

SGA–small for gestational age

SH–shoulder

SI–seriously ill, sacro-iliac

SIB–sibling(s)

SICU–surgical intensive care unit

SIDS–sudden infant death syndrome

SIG–directions for use

SIW–self-inflicted wound

SL–slight(ly)

SLC–short leg cast

SLE–systemic lupus erythematosus

SLR–straight leg raise

SLSLR–side-lying straight leg raise

SLT–sensation to light touch

SWLC–short leg walking cast

SM–small

SMMAI–submaximal multiple angle isometrics

SN–student nurse

SNF–skilled nursing facility

SOB–shortness of breath

SOP–standard operating procedure

S/P–status-post

SPEC–specimen

SPT–static pelvic traction, student physical therapist

SQ–static quadriceps (isometric exercise), subcutaneously

SR–stimulus response

SS–skin score

SSCP–substernal chest pain

SSE–soap suds enema

SSN–social security number

ST–start

STAPH–staphylococcus

STAT–immediately (statim)

STATUS QUO–same condition

STD–sexually transmitted disease

STG–short-term goal(s)

STM–short-term memory

STS–soft tissue swelling

STSG–split-thickness skin graft

SUP–superior, supination, supine

SURG–surgery

SVC–superior vena cava

SVD–spontaneous vaginal delivery

SVT–supraventricular tachycardia

SW–sterile water, social work(er)

SWD–short-wave diathermy

SX–symptom(s)

T

T–temperature, thoracic, trace (muscle test grade)

T1, 2 . . . 12–thoracic spinal levels

T&A–tonsillectomy and adenoidectomy

TAB–tablet

TACHY–tachycardia

TAH–total abdominal hysterectomy

TB–tuberculosis

TBC–total body complaints, tuberculosis culture

TBI–traumatic brain injury

TBSP–tablespoon

TENS–transcutaneous electrical nerve stimulation

TF–tube feeding

TFM–transverse friction massage

TG–triglyceride

TGV–thoracic gas volume

THA–total hip arthroplasty

THR–total hip replacement

TIA–transient ischemic attack

TIB–tibia, tibialis

TIBC–total iron binding capacity

TID–three times daily

TIW–three times a week

TKA–total knee arthroplasty

TKR–total knee replacement

T-L–thoracolumbar

TM–tympanic membrane

TMJ–temporomandibular joint

TNR–tonic neck reflex

TO–telephone order

TP–trigger point

TRACH–tracheostomy

TRAM–treatment rating assessment matrix

TRFD–transferred

TRP–temperature, pulse, respiration

T&S–type and screen

TSH–thyroid stimulating hormone

TT–tetanus toxoid, tilt table

TTN–transient tachypnea of newborn

TTP–tenderness to palpation

TTWB–toe-touch weight bearing

TUR–transurethral resection

TX–traction

U

U/3–upper one third

UA–urinalysis

UBW–usual body weight

UC&S–urine culture and sensitivity

UD–ulnar deviation, unit dose

UE–upper extremity

UMN–upper motor neuron

UNG–ointment

UO–urinary output

URI–upper respiratory infection

US–ultrasound

USN–ultrasonic nebulizer

USP–United States Pharmacopeia

USOH–usual state of health

UT–ureteral catheter

UTI–urinary tract infection
UV–ultraviolet

V

V–vein, void
VA–Veterans Administration
VAG–vagina(l)
VBI–vertebral basilar insufficiency
VC–vital capacity
VD–venereal disease
VE–vaginal examination
VENT–ventilation, ventilator, ventral
VER–visually evoked response
VF–ventricular fibrillation
VFSS–video fluoroscopy swallowing study
VIT–vitamin
VLBW–very low birth weight
VMO–vastus medialis oblique muscle
VMS–variable muscle stimulator
VMT–voluntary muscle test
VO–verbal order
VOL–volume, voluntary, volunteer
VP–ventriculo-parietal (shunt)
VPC–ventricular premature contraction
VS–vital signs, volts per second
VSD–ventricular septal defect
VSI–very seriously ill
VT–ventricular tachycardia
VTX–vertex
VV–varicose veins, veins

W

W–watts, white
W/–with
WB–weight bearing
WBAT–weight bearing as tolerated
WBC–white blood (cell) count
WBQC–wide-based quad cane

WC–wheelchair, work conditioning
W/CM2–watts per centimeter squared
WFE–William's flexion exercises
WFL–within functional limits
WH–work hardening
WIC–women, infants, and children
WK–week
WMS–Wechsler Memory Scale
WNL–within normal limits
WNWD–well-nourished, well-developed
W/O–without
WP–whirlpool
WT–weight, work therapy

X

X–number of repetitions
X RAYS–Roentgen rays

Y

Y–yes
YD–yard
Y/O–year(s) old
YR–year

Special Symbols

≈ –approximately
A –change
Y –female
> –greater than
T –increase
< –less than
D –male
11 –parallel
1° –primary
re./–recheck
2° –secondary
3° –tertiary

Suggested Answer Framework

Chapter 1: Focus on Ethics In this scenario, key primary healthcare professionals responsible for patient B's care seemingly failed to "act in B's best interests," violating the fundamental biomedical ethical principle of beneficence. This breakdown in vital communications between and among providers resulted in B's knee rehabilitation being delayed, with B suffering avoidable pain and stiffness in the affected area associated with that delay. Reflect and share your ideas for systematic improvements in communication to prevent similar adverse events in the future in your practice. This scenario, like Review Case Study #2 in Chapter 1, requires the generation of an incident report for quality management and legal analyses.

Chapter 2: Focus on Ethics From the facts given, C has not breached any patient's privacy, nor has she committed medical record spoliation. C exercised reasonable care by expeditiously noting her documentation error, and exercised reasonable privacy safeguards regarding both D and E by shredding the erroneous blank documentation page from E's record; replacing it with a new blank page; and properly transcribing patient D's medical information into D's record. Keep in mind that not every act of destruction of medical records constitutes the intentional tort (wrong) of record spoliation, as is evident in this case.

Chapter 3: Focus on Ethics This case focuses attention on the multiple dimensions of protection of patient privacy, most of which are reflected in clear, written health professional practice standards. There are eight bases of ethical and legal patient information privacy protection, all of which were violated by R in this scenario: (1) S's constitutional right to information privacy, if this is a federal, state, or municipal public facility;

(2) HIPAA and related federal and state statutory protections for patient PHI (including S's social history); (3) license and/or certification board regulations regarding patient privacy protection; (4) institutional standards regarding confidentiality in S's place of employment; (5) professional association confidentiality ethical standards; (6) judicial case law regarding patient information privacy protection; (7) customary health professional practice standards regarding patient privacy; and (8) personal core ethical and moral values, including the duties of fidelity and truthfulness toward patients under care. For this breach of confidentiality, S potentially faces simultaneous adverse administrative, employment, ethical, and legal actions in multiple venues.

INDEX